★ TAC
FITNESS (40+)
FOUNDATION
REBUILDING

★ FOR BEGINNERS OR ★
RECOVERING FROM INJURY

#1 BEST SELLING FITNESS AUTHOR

STEW SMITH, CSCS, USN (SEAL)

ATTENTION:
A Special Note about how this book was created.

Dear Former Athlete Over 40,

Thank you for claiming your copy of *"Tactical Fitness (40+) – Foundation Rebuilding – For Beginners or Recovering from Injury."*

This book will teach you critical physical rebuilding, recovery and maintenance skills, tools and techniques, and help you rebuild solid habits of fitness that everyday people over 40 need to understand and apply.

This book was originally created as a live interview. Plus, we added exercise pictures, descriptions, links to videos and workouts that focus on all elements of fitness, and allow for proper recovery for the tactical athlete.

That's why Section One reads as a conversation rather than a traditional "book" that talks "at" you. Many find that the conversation really hits home as most of us are not alone in this journey.Section Two and Section Three are more of the traditional fitness book with exercise and workout descriptions / workout charts.

This interview is with who I call the perfect representative for whom this book is made. I also want you to feel as though I am talking "with" you (the reader), much like a coach or a conversion with a friend AND get a world class workout for someone who needs to get back on the fitness wagon.

I felt that creating the material this way would make it fun for you as we discuss these important topics and put them to use quickly, rather than wading through hundreds of pages of why this book is ideal for you.

Get ready to rebuild your fitness and learn how to use recovery methods to feel better and more invigorated each day. Learning how to train effectively to build a fitness foundation and how to actively pursue recovery is the goal of this book.

PS – if you prefer the PDF version, please email me and I will email you the PDF file, as Kindle sometimes has issues centering charts on one page.

Sincerely,

Stew Smith

Table of Contents

Meet Stew Smith

Stew Smith is an expert in Tactical Fitness training, coaching, and writing whose accomplishments include:

Education:

- U.S. Naval Academy Graduate
- Navy SEAL Training Graduate / SEAL Teams (8 years)
- Certified Strength and Conditioning Specialist (CSCS)

Work History:

- Trained thousands of Navy Midshipmen at the Naval Academy
- Trained thousands of military, police, spec ops, and firefighters
- 20+ year history of coaching, training, presenting Tactical Fitness

Awards, Titles, and Designations:

- Amazon Best Selling Fitness Author
- Published Author of Tactical Fitness books and training programs (40)
- Created StewSmith.com 1999
- Created StewSmithFitness.com 2012
- Selling Books since 1998 and eBooks since 2002.
- Online Coaching since 1999

Personal / Business Info:

- Former US Navy SEAL Officer
- Guest instructor at Naval Academy Summer Seminar training 2400 USNA candidates each year for over 20 years.
- Spec Ops Team Coach at the US Naval Academy
- Founder of "Heroes of Tomorrow" which trains military, special ops, police, SWAT, and fire fighters candidates for FREE.
- Created Podcast – Tactical Fitness Report with Stew Smith
- Featured on Fight Science – Special Ops "Ice Man"
- Full time fitness writer (Military.com)

ublished Books Written by Stew Smith

actical Fitness | Tactical Strength | Tactical Mobility
Warrior Workouts – Volume 1
he Complete Guide to Navy SEAL Fitness
Navy SEAL Weight Training Workout
Maximum Fitness
he SWAT Workout
he Special Operations Workout

General Fitness and Nutritional Guides for Everyone

he Beginner / Intermediate Guide to Fitness
Reclaim Your Life - Erin O'Neill Story (beginner / intermediate)
Veterans Fitness - Baby Boomer and a Flat Stomach!
Circuit Training 101 – Beginner / Intermediate Guide to the Gym
he Busy Executive Workout Routine
he Obstacle Course Workout – Prep for Races or Mil, LE, FF
RX / Military Style Workouts – Adding TRX to Military Prep Workouts
Calisthenics and Cardio

The Military / Special Ops Physical Fitness Workouts

Advanced Maintenance / Recovery Plan
he Combat Conditioning Workout
ir Force PJ / CCT Workout
he UBRR – Upper Body Round Robin Workout / Spec Ops version
Navy SEAL Workout Phase 1 | Phase 2 - 3 | Phase 4 Grinder PT
Navy SWCC Workout
rmy Special Forces / Ranger Workout
rmy Air Assault School Workout
rmy Airborne Workout
USMC RECON Workout
USMC OCS / TBS Workout
USMC IST and PFT
he Coast Guard Rescue Swimmer / Navy SAR Workout
he Service Academy Workout (West Point, Navy, Air Force Academy)
he Navy, Air Force, Marine Corp Boot Camp Workout
he Army OCS and PFT Workout
Military, Police, Fire Fighter PT Test Survival Guide
pring / Summer PT / Cardio Cycle
all / Winter Lift Cycle
Increase Strength / Crush the PST / PAST (3:1 Block Periodization Lift Cycle)

The Law Enforcement Physical Fitness Workouts

he FBI Academy Workout | FBI Workout Vol 2
he DEA Workout
he FLETC Workout - Ace the PEB
he PFT Bible: Pushups, Sit-ups, 1.5 Mile Run
he Fire Fighter Workout

Contact Stew Smith (Email, mail)

As part of the downloadable, you do have access to email me at any time and I will answer your questions as soon as possible. Below are the ways to contact me for any of the products and services at www.stewsmith.com.

Mail and email addresses:
StewSmith.com
PO Box 122
Severna Park MD 21146
Email - stew@stewsmith.com

Social Media:

Youtube.com : www.youtube.com/stew50smith (podcasts, swim videos)

Facebook: www.facebook.com/stewsmithfitness (Articles / Q & A)

Instagram: www.instagram.com/stewsmith50 (Cool pics, Motivation)

Twitter: www.twitter.com/stewsmith (Articles, Motivation)

New Podcast:
Tactical Fitness Report with Stew Smith

You can see the podcast on Youtube.com/stew50smith (video),
iTunes and GooglePlay- (search Tactical Fitness Report with Stew Smith), and
Podomatic - For audio version online.

FREE Videos in this Book

In this product, there are free downloadable videos that demonstrate exercises and show techniques in motion by clicking the hyperlinks in the program. These are also on www.youtube.com/stew50smith

As with any generic fitness program, this may not be right for you and you should adjust accordingly if needed. Consulting a physician is recommended before undertaking any new fitness program.

Tactical Fitness Is For Everyone

Tactical Fitness is a relatively new genre of fitness that is primarily designed for people in the military, and police and fire fighter professions where life or death situations occur as part of the job, and fitness can be the determining factor of surviving. However, Tactical Fitness can be for everyone. Consider Tactical Fitness as Functional Fitness for regular LIFE, as well as life or death situations.

If you notice, during emergencies or natural disasters, there are two types of people: Those who need saving and rescuing, and those capable of helping.

We all should have a certain level of tactical / practical fitness that could help us save our own lives or the lives of loved ones in the event of a disaster (natural or man-made). Of course, basic health and wellness cannot be overlooked either. The goal of this book is to help people with the roadmap to being able to save themselves or others in potentially dangerous situations, as well as build healthy habits for the rest of their long lives.

The Tactical Fitness 40+ is a three-phase program (this is phase 1):

Phase 1 – *Tactical Fitness 40+ Foundation Rebuilding*

Phase 2 – *Tactical Fitness 40+ Taking It To The Next Level*

Phase 3 – *Tactical Fitness 40+ Ready to Compete*

And the capstone of the four-part series: <u>Tactical Fitness for the Athlete Over 40: Actively Pursuing Recovery and Healthy Maintenance</u>. The overwhelming positive reaction to this initial advanced program prompted the need for a better progression. Now, the progression is broken up into three phases so the entire spectrum of fitness levels can have a program to rebuild, maintain, and increase physical activity and longevity.

We show you the evolution of the process to go from a low level of fitness and health, to rebuilding the fitness foundation focusing on all the elements of fitness: flexibility, mobility, endurance, stamina, strength, power, speed, and agility. We do this very slowly and progressively with over a year's worth of training in the four programs.

The next section is an interview with a gentleman feeling the struggle of age, health and wellness, mental toughness, and physical performance. We all have these issues at some point.

Chapter One: Stew Smith and the Fitness Foundation

Stew Smith:

[To the reader] Thank you for getting this ebook or book. If you prefer the PDF version of the book and you ordered the printed version or the Kindle, please let me know and I will email it to you, as the PDF tends to be better for the exercise charts in this book. Stew@stewsmith.com

This is a project I've been working on for a while, focusing on the aging athlete. Even though you may not consider yourself "an athlete," I am going to explain how you really are. We are all Tactical Athletes. Because I spent most of my professional writing life creating programs for the 18 to 20-year-old to prepare themselves in tactical fitness for military, law enforcement, and firefighting professions, I started this 20 years ago. And many of my readers that I started writing for back then are now 38 - 40 years old and still in the game. Many have a long history of injuries, and aches and pains that they are trying to fight through, so they can still be active. Many have to start all over again at beginning levels due to a variety of reasons, from illness, injuries, or burnout after 15+ years of war.

This program is for the person who needs to build or rebuild their fitness foundation. I want to introduce you to Gerald Poole. The reason I'm talking with Gerald, is because I think he personifies who I am trying to write for.

There is a segment of the population that I have neglected in my writings. And that's why this whole series is built on people like Gerald. *This is the program for 35, 45, and 50-year-olds, whether you are a civilian, former military, police, or fire service or still active.* Whether you are broken and trying to rebuild, or have been seriously ill and trying to rebuild, or haven't done anything for 20 years and just need to get started again building your fitness foundation—if this is your story—this is your program!

Stew Smith: Gerald has had a unique history of this process, and without me talking about it, let's hear it from him. So, Gerald, welcome. First of all, Gerald thank you for doing this project with me. I think it's really cool that you are going to help me verbalize some issues that are definitely hard to write about. So, let's hear about you. Tell us about your background, your experience in life that's led you to your current position, as well as past fitness histories.

Gerald Poole: I don't have a tremendously intense background when it comes to sports. I would say that I've always been an active person though. In high school, I was a tennis player and a musician for a lot of my high school and college days. I would say physically I was active on the tennis court, and then also in the weight room. I did a lot of weightlifting, typically bodybuilding workouts three times a week, and then cardio workouts three times a week. Now, I'm 43. So, when I talk about high school and college, you can kind of figure out how long ago that may have been. I was never too intense with any one physical activity. When I talk about the bodybuilding workouts, those types of workouts, at least in my opinion, are obviously good for you. Lifting weights, building muscle, getting leaner, increasing bone density, and increasing your cardio are all great. But it was mostly done for *aesthetics*, especially when I was younger. Everyone wants to get bigger muscles and things like that. That was my true foundation.

Stew Smith: Okay. So, you have a decent fitness foundation. What would you say about your friends? Your workout partners, your teammates? How are they doing in comparison to you? Along this journey, you maybe had workout partners, or you have friends and mentors that you've met along your fitness journey.

Gerald Poole: That has changed over the years. Now, what I'm looking for is functionality, and being capable of doing things because I am fit. And when you talk about some of my friends, and some of the events I've done, transitioning from that bodybuilding aesthetics kind of mindset to more functionality and capability ... I went from training for aesthetics to saying, "How can I get tougher? How can I be someone who isn't going to quit when things get hard? How can I become somebody that really trains hard, and then goes, okay, well, this was a nice 40-minute workout, but how can I handle four more hours?"

So, when you ask about the people that I've been hanging out with, that is an important part of becoming more mentally tough, and more capable at endurance events. Surrounding myself with like-minded people was important, even though it's hard to find people like that in your immediate circle of friends. That mindset is not as common as you would hope it to be. So, I started turning to online sources for learning how to think that way. And a lot of that had to do with watching your videos, or other Navy SEAL videos, reading GORUCK stories, and certain books by special operators, and things like that.

So, I really went from hanging out with people who wanted to get big in the gym, to people seeking something different from their training.

Stew Smith: I know exactly what you are talking about, but you know what? I think many people are lying if they don't say that was probably what got them in the weight room in the first place.

Stew Smith: I was 14 years old. It was a contest. How much you could bench. When I was growing up, it was Joe Weider workout books, in the 80s. Three sets of eight, and do a couple of exercises, and I thought I was done with a workout. Things evolve, and things change along with your goals and with your desires. So, what is your goal now? Let's talk about a short-term goal of one to two years, and then let's talk about a long-term goal at age 50 plus.

Gerald Poole: I think I'll start by saying ... For me, this became the journey to becoming more mentally tough. And why is that important? Why did I want to do that? What significance did it have for me?

In my early 30s, I was thinking, "I've got to be capable of doing more." I want to be able to look back on things that I've done, whether it was last week, or 20 years ago, or whatever, and say, "I did really hard things, and I hung in there." I want to become my best self. I want to know that when things got hard, I didn't quit.

I started getting interested in reading about Navy SEALs. And there are some Navy SEAL camps, and military-inspired events out there. And I thought, "How cool would it be to do these events?" And even though I hate to say this, I've got to be honest. I failed.

Stew Smith: You know, they are good gut checks.

Gerald Poole: I failed...

Stew Smith: They are tough gut checks. You are talking about Mark Divine's program right?

Gerald Poole: Yes.

Stew Smith: Great guy. Great gut check. Great challenge.

Gerald Poole: Yeah. Great challenge. And as embarrassing as it is to talk about, it's very real. I think you need to talk about what's real to get better. I do not want to sugar-coat things and make excuses for why things didn't work. I must be honest with myself.

Stew Smith: But before you do, though, let's talk about this. Your foundation was gym workouts, aesthetics, maybe 30, 45-minute workouts. Something longer?

Gerald Poole:	Yes.
Stew Smith:	And then you say, "Alright, I'm going to do this. I'm going to start focusing on these tougher events as mental toughness challenges." And so that's where I talk a lot about tactical fitness. And it really does depend on your fitness foundation before you start attempting some of these hard challenges. The transition from this fitness foundation of power lifting or weightlifting or other sports into these harder challenges may take a good year or more. This is what I tell tactical athletes that are trying to be military, law enforcement, and firefighters.

However, the reason you are being interviewed here is because you are my tactical athlete, personified, for civilian purposes. And what I mean by that is ... We all need to be tactical athletes. And maybe we call them "functional athletes," or "functional fitness," or whatever. There are so many terms to describe what I'm trying to say. But, basically, it is this: When there's an accident that happens, there are two types of people. There are people that need to be saved, and there are people who are doing the saving. |
Gerald Poole:	Right.
Stew Smith:	And I have been a big proponent of having a good fitness foundation and abilities, so that when something happens, I can be the helper. So, when something goes down, I want to be able to be the guy who can save my family, save a victim from whatever circumstance, or myself for that matter. Having the confidence that my physical ability can save lives is a huge mental boost that not many people have. The lack of this type of confidence can detour people from accepting new challenges and bettering themselves as well. It spills over into other areas of your life too.
Gerald Poole:	Right.
Stew Smith:	When we talk about tactical fitness, I want people to realize that it's not just for military, law

enforcement, or firefighters. ***It's really for everybody.*** And I wanted to share that with you, because after talking with you for a while, I realized this is what you were trying to do.

Gerald Poole: One hundred percent. And that's exactly right. I don't want to be just a muscle head. I want to be capable when something happens. Because today, I think it is very relevant.

Unfortunately, you turn on the news, and you see crazy things happening every day, either natural or man-made disasters. Or, what if one of my kids falls into a swimming pool? Am I going to be able to jump in there and get him without getting into trouble myself? I think being a tactical athlete is more relevant to civilians than most civilians even believe or would begin to imagine. I think it's very relevant.

And it doesn't have to be a catastrophic event. It doesn't have to be me trying to save my wife from tragedy or getting the kids out of the house in a fire. I have a two-year-old and a five-year-old. It can just be both wanting to be carried at the same time and being able to do that.

Stewart Smith: Yeah. There you go.

Gerald Poole: And that happens a lot. I am always carrying them. And you talk about aging athletes ... At 43 and well into my 50's and 60's, I want to be rolling with them still.

Stew Smith: Yeah. That's a good one.

Gerald Poole: And I think the tactical mindset and being a tactical athlete will enable me to do that.

Stew Smith: Absolutely. What about some of the things you have done? Whenever you started on this journey with these tactical fitness challenges, what were some of the events that you did? What made you re-circle and come about attacking these in a different way?

Gerald Poole: So, that's really, for me, the crux of this. We mentioned SEALFIT, and Mark Divine's camps early on. And again, being honest with myself is hard. But I think you have to be honest in order to get better, and you have to realize the strength in saying, "Hey, I can't be satisfied with failing. I need to confront what I did wrong, and I need to figure out how to fix it, and I need to move forward."

So, when I was in my early 30s and I wanted to try some of these things, like SEALFIT, I still had the mentality of training like a bodybuilder. And I was thinking, "Hey, wouldn't it be cool to go through the SEALFIT camp? Wouldn't it be cool to *tell* somebody I did that?" **Those are not the right reasons to do something that difficult.** It's garbage to think, "Oh, I want to do this so I can *tell* someone I did it." So I trained for the SEALFIT camp by doing bodybuilding workouts three times a week and cardio three times a week for 40 minutes to an hour each session. I failed miserably. It was bad. I quit. I just quit.

Stew Smith: I tell people all the time, man ... There's no 30, 40-minute workout that's going to prepare you for a day of Spec-Ops training, and I think that was your first issue. But, you really do have to put in the time to training like this. When you say you failed, what happened? Was it a physical breakdown? Was it being cold, wet and miserable? Mentally challenging? When you say you failed, what happened?

Gerald Poole: Great questions. I actually quit twice—on two separate occasions— and for very different reasons. The first reason was I just had no clue what I was getting into. I had no clue at all. I was under-prepared from a physical and a mental standpoint. I just had no idea. I had no idea about the intensity, about the pacing. I had no idea about the types of exercises. I thought a plank hold for anything more than 30 seconds was impossible and that people did not do such things.

I was just not prepared at all. And I think I made it through about six hours the first time. A lot of it was mental, and I just didn't understand that. I think maturity and emotional intelligence are critical in developing your mental toughness.

So, a year came and went, and I tried again. The second time I quit right before I even started and it was for a different reason, mainly anxiety. I realized that I lacked maturity, emotional awareness and emotional intelligence.

I've had a hard time controlling fear in my life. I would have all of these ideas in my head about what I wanted to accomplish, or what I wanted to achieve. And it would seem so clear. Then, I would go to execute, and it would just fall apart because of that anxiety.

Also, that second time around at the SEALFIT camp, all of these Crossfit guys were there, some of the best Crossfit guys in the world. I showed up, and I'm like, *"I'm not going to be able to hang with these guys. This is modeled after Hell Week. It's modeled after being a good team member, about pulling your weight, about helping your team. I'm not going to be able to help these guys. I'm going to be a liability."* So, right off the bat, that type of thinking got into my head, and I just was like, "*Don't even try to hang with these guys.*"

Stew Smith: That is when you have to stop listening to yourself and start TALKING to yourself – just positively.

Gerald Poole: And so those are really two different reasons at two different attempts of why I tried and I quit. And so, this was in my early 30s. And I kind of resigned to the fact that, *"This isn't for you."* However, we talk about having powerful WHYS and I have a totally different set of WHYS now at 43 years old.

So those ideas—the ideas of being able to get through tough challenges—went dormant for several years, and then I started getting that itch again in my late 30s. And the reason why is because I got married, and I had kids. And my WHYS—what kind of Dad I wanted to be—shaped why I started getting back into this and saying, *"No, no, no, you **CAN** do this. You just have to take a different approach."*

Stew Smith:

There you go. Yeah. You know what? WHYS, they come in all different sized packages. Some people's "WHY" is just because they like the adrenaline rush. For some it's, *"I want to do it because I can show people I can do it, and show them they are wrong for doubting me."* There is no good or bad why, I think.

But what you went through, there is a huge roadblock that I think many people today have. Most people probably wouldn't even consider attempting what you've done, or what you tried to do. But I think there is a very big group that is in that zone of, *"I'd like to do that, but I'm not sure how I could prepare for it. I'm not sure if I'm capable of doing that."*

But I will say this, and I tell this to everybody, your body is ten times stronger than your mind will ever let it be, if that makes sense.

Gerald Poole:

Absolutely. Yes.

Stew Smith:

If you can disengage that little part of your brain, especially the anxiety before an event, the pain of going through the event, all those little things that make us say we want to stop, you will one day realize that your body is ten times stronger than your mind will let it be. And you have to think about this, our brain is built to keep our body alive, and survive. These are natural survival thoughts, and techniques, and skills that your brain has come up with through the eons to keep you alive. Your brain saying, "No, you better not do this, that's stupid," is there to keep you alive.

Gerald Poole: Right.

Stew Smith: It's unbelievable what your body can do. So, what I try to do, and I think what a lot of these programs try to do, is try to tap into that part of the brain that is going to give you some unbelievable abilities, physically, but also some confidence into handling anything that comes your way in the future. Whether that is having to stay up all night to get a job done, whatever that task is, it is amazing what some of these programs do for you. And I admire you for trying it, and I admire you for turning around and trying it again.

You got through this roadblock. What's next for you?

Gerald Poole: Yeah. So, good commentary on that, because I think you hit on something just now, and also I think you've talked about this in your podcast, and it is that whole idea of mental toughness. I became obsessed with it. What does it mean, this elusive concept of being mentally tough? And you watch videos of Special Ops guys and say, "That level of fitness is something that I will never be able to possess." Or, "That's something that I can't understand." I think we sell ourselves short with how much potential we have with, *"Becoming mentally tough."*

Some people might just get it right off the bat and be super mentally tough, and not have to go through this process. But for me it was being exposed to difficult things incrementally, and having little victories. I think you mentioned that in one of your podcasts, the concept of, "Finding the fuel when the tank is empty," and "Getting comfortable being uncomfortable." Both are so true when trying to define mental toughness.

Further, it started with me thinking, *"Look. I have two kids that I want to not just take care of as babies and children, but I want to raise them to be certain kinds of adults."* And I want them to be kind people. I want them to be capable people. I want them to be adjusted. I want them to be strong. Because, there are a lot of fragile people out there, and I _don't_ want to be one of them. I don't want my kids to be either. I don't want, when something gets hard, for them to go, *"Oh, I can't do it,"* or *"I'm going to quit." Because life is going to be full of difficulty.*

Stew, I started believing, *"I've got to go back and finish these things I started,"* because I can't teach my kids these types of concepts if I don't do the same things. I can't teach them to never quit if I've been a quitter. I can't teach them to do difficult things if I don't do difficult things.

We talk about these military-inspired events. So, I looked into doing a GORUCK. I started with a GORUCK Light, three or four years ago. And I wasn't in the right kind of shape, or the shape I'm in now, or the shape I will be two years from now. But doing that gave me a taste of, *"All right. Let's do something challenging on a smaller scale."* That's a short-term, smaller goal that I can achieve, get that patch (when you complete an event, a patch is earned), and say, *"Okay. I can start building my way up from this to more difficult events."*

And the most recent event I did that I'm pretty proud of was the GORUCK Mogadishu Mile HTL – a 24 hour Heavy, a 12 hour Tough, and a 6 hour Light together, all back to back to back over a weekend. I think I slept for an hour, maybe two. It was tough.

Stew Smith: Damn. That's awesome. GORUCK, by the way - I have to give a plug to GORUCK, because they do such a great job, not only with their great backpacks, but their events. Their events are really life changing for people.

Gerald Poole:	Absolutely. Aside from doing a 5K or a Turkey Fun Run or something like that, this gives you the opportunity to start pushing yourself on a smaller scale. The Lights are shorter. They're not necessarily easier. But you put on your rucksack, you carry a certain amount of weight in it, and you travel a certain distance with a team carrying heavy things and doing PT along the way.
Stew Smith:	Getting comfortable being uncomfortable one step at a time.
Gerald Poole:	Yes! And it's something I think about a lot. So, in any case, I finished this event. Some of the people there could run circles around me doing PT. And one of these guys was just amazing. He was over 50. You see all these people coming together of varying ages and backgrounds, and you think, *"These are NOW my people and workout partners and motivational friends."* They get it and these events started giving me goals and things to look forward to, which also generated an amazing amount of happiness for me.
	The biggest take away for me was, *"I can do things that are difficult."* I would've failed this GORUCK HTL had I not started incrementally and built myself up to it over time. And so, now I want to get to the point where I can go back to Mark Divine's camp and get through it. And that's one of my long-term goals. And there are a couple of other things I want to try, as well.
Stew Smith:	Nice.
Gerald Poole:	This last event—the Mogadishu Mile HTL—was six weeks ago, and I lost toenails, had blisters and it hurt. Just taking steps became excruciating. But, it was one of those things where I thought, *"Don't quit, because this event will be over. Your feet will heal. But if you quit, you're never going to be able to redeem yourself."* And so, as painful as it was, I kept moving. And when I was finished with that, I was changed, transformed if you will.

Stew Smith:	Nice. I think, in there, somewhere, you discovered what mental toughness is. There's a hard-to-find definition. Some people will say, *"You want mental toughness? Just start getting tougher,"* *which is a great, simplistic way of looking at it.* *But there's some mystery behind it too, such as, "Finding the fuel when the tank is empty."* I think that is a unique definition for what mental toughness is. And it is pure heart and will. You willed yourself to be able to do that.
Gerald Poole:	Absolutely. And I think I had been overcomplicating it for quite some time. Mental toughness is not in some motivational quote. It's not some complicated recipe. It's getting comfortable being uncomfortable in increments increasingly more difficult, and building on that thought of, *"Hey, I stuck with this.* *Next time, I'm going to do something even more difficult."*
Stew Smith:	And that's no joke, man. Let me just tell you something. That Mogadishu Mile is very similar to the exact same type of training we put our candidates through to prepare them for SEAL training. Because there's a little thing they used to call Mini-BUDS that you would go through. And it's basically a 36-hour "Heck Day." So instead of a 120-hour Hell Week that you're going to endure at your fourth week of SEAL training, it's a 36-hour version of that.

And people come to terms with a lot of things. *"Do I really want to do this in my future?"* And many people come back but many do not. And then they have to progress a little more to find their weaknesses in these things.

I think that's where you're starting to see your success. You've acknowledged some weaknesses. You've addressed them. You've tested them through these challenges, and now those weaknesses aren't so much weaknesses anymore. They are now borderline strengths. Because we all come to the table with certain strengths and weaknesses. And I think it is mainly through |

	honesty and maturity that you have to realize this to move forward.
Gerald Poole:	Absolutely.
Stew Smith:	I think you're doing that. I love your term, you were "Overcomplicating things."
Gerald Poole:	I think people sell themselves short and they overcomplicate it. It really becomes just doing it. But it's acknowledging where you are as well. If you're someone who's never exercised before, and you're 20 pounds overweight, and you're sitting on the couch, and thinking, *"Geez, it would be cool to do something like that and challenge myself, but I couldn't do it,"* you're mistaken! You can do it! It's just that you have to start incrementally, and you have to build upon each tiny little victory until you can say, *"Okay, I'm going to set that goal to do a GORUCK Light in six months,"* or whatever it is.
Stew Smith:	And the journey's different for everybody.
Gerald Poole:	Exactly.
Stew Smith:	The journey to get there is going to be different for everybody, with their logical progressions to prepare for these types of events.
Gerald Poole:	Many people don't realize that, at least I didn't. I thought, "Well, if I'm not mentally tough right off the bat, if I can't go finish this camp, then it's just not for me." That's wrong.
Stew Smith:	Yes. In fact, in military terms, these events are called *"Stress inoculations."* And they start off with you getting up out of bed, early, before work, when you are probably at the most comfortable you will ever be in a day. Let's face it, there's nothing more comfortable than being on a pillow with covers over you, lying in bed. And then you hear that alarm go off at 4:30, or 5:30 in the morning and that is a very uncomfortable feeling. The

comfortable version is to go push that snooze button, or turn the alarm off, and just stay in bed.

The uncomfortable version is getting up and making that a habit. And then, that is kind of the beginning of this stress inoculation. The next step is getting out of the house and going for a run. Or jumping in a swimming pool. It's never warm when you do that, first thing in the morning. That's probably one of the hardest things for me. I dip my toe in the pool and say *"This is going to suck."* But you jump in anyway. It takes about a hundred meters for the cold to wear off.

All these little things are just little stress inoculations that, like you were saying, "It is building you up to be a more mentally tough, resilient person." To be able to handle any future stress that comes about.

Stew Smith: And another thing, too, you mentioned - seeing that 50-year-old guy in there kicking butt. That has always motivated me. When I see guys older than me doing it, and getting it done, I say, *"All right. I like this. This is really good."* Because I think there are a lot of benefits to seeing something in order for you to believe it's true. There's a saying, *"You have to see it to believe it."*

Gerald Poole: Right.

Stew Smith: And when you can see people finishing these events, you can say, "I can do that. He's 20 years older than me. I should be able to do that."

There are training programs that can get you to that level – this is one of many I have created. They work if you do them. This is all about learning. I think some humility in there is very key. It's always good to keep learning. These are processes to get you to that next level. I am still learning every day and trying out new programs.

Gerald Poole: The humility part—getting rid of the ego. That was such a big deal for me. Yes, I know I failed. I quit. I quit twice. I have to acknowledge that and say, "It's okay, because I'm turning things around. I'm going back to finish what I started," or *"I'm learning how not to quit."* And I couldn't have gotten to this place unless I had gone through the failures and the quitting, and subsequently the desire to get back up there and finish some of these things.

So, I think ego can be a big, big roadblock to achieving things. And I think it's important to start from wherever you are. Treat yourself like a beginner, like you say. You don't have to be happy with where you are, but you can accept it and be content in thinking, "Okay, I have to start somewhere. I can't be an excellent athlete until I'm an intermediate athlete."

One more thing that you were talking about when you mentioned the programs you have written. So, I've tried a bunch of different programs. And a lot of them, if not all of them, are military based, predominantly Special Operations or SEAL-based training regimens. And there are a lot of great ones out there.

However, for me that was the problem, that there were so many sources. Which one do I choose? The reason I gravitated towards you was because the programming became specific to me as a person. I wasn't getting a prefab email of, *"Here. Here's what you need to do today."* Which ... and again, a lot of these programs are good, but what's unique about yours is that the programming's specific to the individual.

And so that's why I gravitated towards you. Because you make the training regimen for me each week, and not only is it specific to what I did last week, it's specific to my individual goals as well. It's also tailored to my age. It's tailored to whatever injuries I may be dealing with or trying to prevent, and you take the time to say, *"Hey, look, we have to talk at least each weekend, so each week when I make your new program, I can make sure that it's a logical progression from what you did last time."*

Stew Smith: Yes. That is what we do. And it does work. I've been doing it for almost 20 years, long before people really thought there was an internet business. But, like I said, I find that your story, where you have come from, and where you are now, and where you want to go, is ideal for taking it to the next level. Because you had a foundation coming in, and you've built upon that foundation. And now it's time for you to move on from the aches and pains of previous challenges, and build upon, and ... Let's take it to the next level!

So, for me, especially for the guy over 40, and myself too, periodization programming has been a lifesaver. It's the way I have arranged these workouts throughout the year to progressively work through ALL the elements of fitness: strength, power, muscle stamina, endurance, speed and agility, and mobility and flexibility. You're in a cycle right now where, we're trying to build more work capacity. We're kind of pushing some of the longer workouts, working on some endurance. But, there's going to be a time when we need to pull back from that, and work on some strength training. Work on some foundation training, foundation of strength. And that's going to help you be able to endure some of the harder elements in future events that you do.

And that's the periodization programming that I've been doing for 20 years, and I really think it's saved my life. And then the other thing that has saved me has been that after 40 years old, I started adding in a mobility day once a week. And that is one of the keys to this program, as well. I'm making this program to rebuild the foundation, and even for taking it to the next level. And then the third phase of this program is going to be, *"I'm ready to compete, and go after it."*

Gerald Poole: That's what I like about working with you. It could be mid-week and I might think, *"I need a mobility day,"* and we rearrange. Also, one of the best things I have learned is getting in the pool in chest-deep water and doing dynamic stretches. I'd never heard of that before and I didn't know how valuable it would be. You also talk about foam rolling and stretching, too. But getting into the water, into chest-deep water, and doing dynamic stretches has been the most helpful thing in terms of recovery that I hadn't been doing before.

Stew Smith:
Oh, it has saved me. Like I said, I've been doing it now for almost eight years. And I just started writing about it about four years ago, just because I wanted to really make sure it was working. I always test things out for a couple of years before I write about it. And that's with any workout that I do. But this one, I had to share. And now I'm putting it in all workouts, even for the 22-year-old guy who probably doesn't even need it. I've seen performance gains the following two or three workouts after a mobility day that typically hadn't been happening, all because of the addition of this little "active rest" day.

Because here's what happens if you put a mobility day in the middle of your week. Let's say you hit it hard Monday and Tuesday. And you have a Wednesday mobility day. Well, normally, that would've been a hard Wednesday workout, and then a hard Thursday workout, and a hard Friday workout. And by Friday and Saturday, your workouts are just horrible. You have no juice left, and you're really getting by on fumes. I've seen such a big change, not only in myself as the aging athlete, but in my younger athletes as well. They take this midweek mobility day that helps to create killer performances on Friday and Saturday, which they were lacking before.

Gerald Poole:
Right. And they end their week on a high note with that amazing workout, because they had the opportunity to have an active recovery day, which is also key for injuries too, because I have three herniated discs. I have a torn disc. I have bone spurs. My lumbar area is a mess. And I have to work with that. I figured out a way to work with it,

and these mobility days help me do that. I think they not only help give my body that active recovery it needs, but they also help with some of the injuries that I'm dealing with, while making some of the other harder workouts possible.

Stew Smith: Yeah. I love it. So, let's just change topic a little bit, and just talk about recovery and maintenance a little more. Is your life stressful? How would you describe your life? You have a normal, stressful life? Do you have stress in your life?

Gerald Poole: Yes. Absolutely. I've worked really hard at being better at dealing with anxiety and it has made me more powerful. I know that sounds weird. But if you can harness some of those stressors, and overcome them, you can become stronger. So yes, the initial stress of being an anxious person, my career, my goals and two very young kids can all add up. Also, good stress is still stress.

Additionally, I've been training jiu-jitsu for a long time, and I want to get to class a couple of times a week. So trying to fit in all of this training, getting the kids to school, making sure they get to bed, trying to make sure they get their teeth brushed. I mean everything!

It would be easy to say, *"I don't have time."* I've heard people say that, and I get it, but then you'll hear, *"Well, you need to make time."* And it's just that simple.

Stew Smith: Yes. I love it. So, obviously, everybody's life is stressful. I asked that in a joking manner. But you are relieving your stress through these activities, now.

Gerald Poole: Aside from being a father, and enjoying my family, I would say that training is "my thing." It's more than a hobby to me. It's more of a lifestyle. It is, aside from being a father, the single biggest source of happiness for me. Knowing that I've failed all of these things and decided I wasn't going to give up is an awesome feeling! It brings me a tremendous source of, not just stress relief, but happiness as well.

Stew Smith: Very good point. So, here's another thing, too. When your life is stressful, and all of ours are, there's no getting around that. Sometimes the last thing you ever want to do on that very stressful day is a butt-kicking workout that's going to stress you out even more, physically. But after a very stressful day, doing something challenging for 15, 20 minutes is great. It's a great way to get those fight/flight hormones out of your body. It will help to metabolize them through some activity.

Then, you go through a nice, steady, relaxing breathing cycle. It could be as gentle as a walk. It could be a nice, easy jog or low impact cardio, to get the parasympathetic nervous system going again, while breathing deeply. Deep breathing, meditation, easy cardio, and getting more oxygen into your body is a great way to metabolize stress hormones.

Where a lot of people go wrong, is they either do one of two things. They either don't do anything, which is bad, or they just crush it in the weight room, and add more stress to their central nervous system on top of all the daily stress that they're putting into their lives. And it's harder to recover from that.

Stew Smith: Once again, there's always a tangible aspect to training. But then there are intangible aspects to training that are very difficult to get to unless you put in the time.

Gerald Poole: That's right. If mental toughness has a lot to do with flexing that mental muscle, some of the only times you can do that is when you're doing something you don't want to do, or something difficult. When I'm halfway through a difficult workout, and still have a long way to go, and I'm weak, and I'm not feeling like I want to do it, I know that's a critical time for me to practice flexing that mental muscle. I also know that I have to be accountable to myself and to you, so that keeps me going. Also, thinking about how good it will feel to get through it and not quit helps a lot.

Stew Smith: Absolutely. I would say one of my biggest jobs training young people who want to go into these professions—especially the Special Ops professions—is not just coming up with great workouts that build them and prepare them for what their future task is. It's also about pulling the reins on them and saying, "No, you don't need to do that. Why don't you take a recovery day today instead of preparing for a 50-mile racing event? Let's pull back."

Gerald Poole: Right.

Stew Smith: Because, I have seen it happen way too many times. Guys that are hard chargers push and push and push and push, and then something breaks. In fact, that's why I even wrote the first Tactical Fitness For the Athlete Over 40 book. And it's my own story. My own story was me breaking down at age 28 after years of training ridiculously hard. And I had a lot of success. However, that success came at a price. In the end, that success bit me. So now, I teach people that you need to learn how to start training for longevity, in addition to being smart about the stress you're accumulating every day.

Gerald Poole: Right. And that has a lot to do with removing that ego.

Stew Smith: Yes.

Gerald Poole: And it's especially difficult for me, Stew, because I'm someone who's trying to come back from failures. And when you're trying to come back from failures, and you're dedicated to your goals, you want to make sure you're pushing really hard. And it's really difficult to differentiate between, *"You need a mobility day, you need a rest day,"* and, *"No, you've got to get out there and get it done. Even if you have to crawl through it, you have to get it done."*

I have to learn how to take a day that wasn't programmed and make it a mobility day when it's clearly needed.

Stew Smith: Yes. Absolutely. I think we all do. I would say that every week I try to do a mobility day. There may be a week, one week out of the month, where I skip it and move on. And that's okay if you want to do it. But then I make sure the next week I don't skip it. And some weeks, we will do this really hard weekend workout. But I make sure when we come back on Monday, we do a mobility day. And then we get a couple good workouts in and on Friday, we do another mobility day. So, sometimes there are actually times when two mobility days in one week makes sense. It just depends on how much you're crushing it.

Gerald Poole: Yeah. And there are many unique things that you'll put into a mobility day that are very helpful.

Stew Smith: Absolutely, I agree with everything you're doing. Your WHYS, I think, are not only just fun challenges to get you to these events, and accomplish some things that you want to accomplish, but they're also going to help you with your ability to be the guy who can help people. I want you to know, this is what I think it should come down to for all of us: the ability to be able to help people, as well as yourself. Because there are those times when you have to be able to help yourself too.

Also, don't forget that fitness is a journey, and not a destination. There's no, **"Okay, I'm done. I've reached my _____."** Like you said, it is a hobby or a lifestyle. Experiment with different programs. Learn how to train. Learn how to cycle through different elements of fitness. And we're talking about all the elements of fitness. We're talking about endurance. Strength. Muscle stamina. Flexibility. Mobility. Speed and agility. **Periodization Training!** All of those things are elements that we need to be better tactical athletes. We have to be good at all of them. There can't be one that we cannot do, and still be considered a ready tactical athlete.

For instance, if you can't swim, you are ineffective on 75% of this earth, which is a horrible thing to think about. And there are many people who cannot swim. Take a lesson at a local YMCA. Take a beginner kids' lesson if you need to. There's nothing wrong with just getting an instructor, and learning how to swim.

Gerald Poole: Also, it helps to know that people like you (Navy SEALs) struggle with things too. It's easy to think certain people don't have flaws or weaknesses and are good at everything. But I started learning that, no; everybody has things they need to work on. Everybody has things they want to improve upon. Everybody has things they've failed. And as soon as you start realizing that, it helps make daunting goals seem more achievable.

It's something that we all face. I am not unique in that I have failed. I am not unique in that I need to lose 20 pounds and get off the couch.

And when you talk about helping people, I think that's another source of happiness as well. I think kindness is so underrated.

Stew Smith: Well, I will say this. I think we've hit all the things I wanted to hit on in this conversation. Now, the rest of this project—as you read on—will be exercises and workouts, arranged in a way where I'm going to phase this thing out. And this one's for beginners. And we're going to rebuild you if you are injured, and we're going to focus on all the different elements of fitness. It may take some time, but be patient. I promise you, a year from now, you will wish you had started today!

Gerald Poole: Absolutely. And like you said, it's a journey. It's a succession of successful workouts. A succession of successful days. A succession of successful weeks and months. It's not going to happen tomorrow, but accept that, and have fun with it.

And that's really what's brought me happiness. I may not even be halfway there! I'm excited to know that I'm going to go back and crush my goals, and that I'm going to be so much more fit a year from now, and two years from now. And yeah, I'm anxious to achieve my goals, but it might take another two years. It might take ... I don't know how long! I don't care. It's the process that I've really started to focus on, and fall in love with.

Stew Smith:

There you go. I love that. Because, do what you like to do first. Whatever gets you into the weight room. Whatever gets you into the gym. Whatever exercise. You like to bench-press? Make sure bench-press is a part of your workout. You love to bench-press? Do it.

But then start adding some supplemental training to help balance out what you like and what gets you into the weight room. Also work your lower body. Work your upper back. Work your core. Work your cardio. All of those things. Otherwise it makes this journey a little more difficult. There are many things I like, but didn't like before, because I'd never tried them. You have to go try it. See if you like it.

Stew Smith:

Give it a shot. Next thing you know, you're going to be on this new journey. And it might be triathlons. It might be marathons. It might be GORUCK challenges. It might be the SEALFIT challenge. It might be one of our Special Ops Triathlons. Whatever those goals are that you have can grow from getting into the weight room and building persistence every day. A little bit of motivation at first evolves into habits that you've created. And when you can't rely on your motivation, what do you rely on?

Gerald Poole:

Your discipline.

Stew Smith:

Discipline. You have disciplined yourself through all these persistent daily challenges, and when you don't feel like training you can say, *"Well, I'm not really motivated to work out, but I'm going to go work out anyway."*

Gerald Poole:	Exactly!

Stew Smith: Absolutely. There are many times I don't feel like getting up at 5:15 and working out with guys 20 years younger. But, I know I'll always feel better after doing it. And that's the key. So, Gerald, I want to thank you so much for your time. Because, like I said, your story is so common. There are many people out there from all types of backgrounds that share the same goal of being tactically fit and having the ability to provide assistance if needed, or just to be able to help themselves.

Stew Smith: One day, I want you to say—and to anybody who's reading this—"My fitness level saved my life." Do not let it be the reason you die, or the reason you were unable to help someone you love. That's how important fitness is. And that's what tactical fitness is all about.

Stew Smith: **<u>Now let's get to work!</u>**

Getting Started

The following stretching plan will assist you with getting started again safely and without as much post-exercise soreness.

Most injuries are strains or muscle pulls that can be prevented with a few simple stretching exercises done daily. The added flexibility will not only assist in injury prevention, but with speed workouts and help you to run faster. The following is a stretching routine that can be used whether you are a beginner or advanced athlete.

The Warm-Up Routine

Finding what works best for you as a warm-up is critical to your success in fitness testing and long-term job performance. Increasing your flexibility should be the first goal before starting fitness/athletic activity. This dynamic stretch routine is a quick and effective way to warm up prior to your workout, as well as cooldown in the pool afterwards to produce the desired results of mobility and flexibility.

Chapter Four: Dynamic Stretching and Core Exercises

A quick and easy to follow dynamic stretching routine will demonstrate the way to warm up and prepare for workouts. Take 5-10 minutes and get warmed up with these leg movements prior to working out. You can do this one on land (typically) or add a session in chest deep water. Click the hyperlink to see most of these in motion.

Jog or Bike - 5 minutes **Butt Kickers - 1 minute** **Frankenstein Walks - 1 minute** **Bounding in Place - 1 minute** **Side Steps with hip opener – 1 min** **Leg Swings Front / Back– 1 minute** **Leg Swings (Left / Right) – 1 minute** **Calf/Shin Warm-up – 1 minute** **Burpees – 1 minute** **Light Arm Shoulder Chest Stretch** **Light Thigh Stretch** **Light Hamstring Stretch** **Back Roll** **Light ITB Roll** **Shin Roll**

Warming Up for Workouts

Jog, walk, or bike five minutes or do a series of light calisthenics like jumping jacks, crunches, push-ups, squats prior to stretching. Dynamic stretching is a major part of warming up prior to any athletic movements. To reduce muscle fatigue and soreness and prevent injuries, perform a good warm-up using these dynamic/static stretches. You can also use these on the back end of a hard workout to cool-down from hard activity as well.

Jog or Bike 5 minutes – Get the blood flowing.

<u>Butt Kickers</u> - **1 minute:** Jog slowly and flex your hamstrings to pull your heels to your butt on each step. Do with knees down and knees up for 30-60 seconds.

<u>Frankenstein Walks</u> - **1 minute:** Walk and kick high each step. Try to kick your hands in front of you. Do 10 kicks with each leg.

ounding - 1 minute: Do high powered skipping for 1 minute. Start off with gular skipping then lift knees high each step. Do in place for 1 minute or cross a 50-100-yard field.

ide steps - 30 seconds each direction: Work lateral movement into the arm-up. Mix in a few squats with cross-overs. Do for 1 minute back and forth each direction.

alf/Shin Warm-up – 1 minute: Alternate lifting heels off the floor and toes off e floor. This is a shins/calves builder to help strengthen legs for nning/rucking.

Burpees – 1 minute: Drop into the pushup position. Quickly drop your chest to the floor and back to the up position. Bring your feet up and stand and jump 4-6 off the ground to finish the rep.

Light Arm Shoulder/Chest stretch: Pull your arm across your torso to stretch rear/deltoid and trapezius region. Then pull your arms backward as far as you can to stretch the chest/front shoulder connections.

Thigh Stretch – Standing: - Standing, bend your knee and grab your foot at the ankle. Pull your heel to your butt and push your hips forward. Hold for 10-15 seconds and repeat with the other leg.

Hamstring Stretch #1 and #2: - From the standing position, bend forward at the waist and come close to touching your toes, slightly bend your knees and pull your torso closer to your legs. Go back and forth from straight legs to bent knees to feel the top/bottom part of the hamstring stretch. You should feel this stretching the back of your thighs.

For more Static Stretches – See Link:

http://site.stewsmithptclub.com/StaticStretches.pdf

<u>Myofascial Release</u> – Learn this term and get a foam roller for yourself. See
<u>Foam Roller Article / Video</u>

This coupled with cooldowns or mobility days will make all the difference in the world with your recovery from tough workouts.

<u>Back roll:</u> Sit on foam roller and move slowly back and forth as you lie on the roller. Move your legs to move your body over the roller. Do for 1-2 minutes each body part.

<u>ITB roll:</u> Lay on your side in a side plank position and place foam roller under your hip. Move forward and roll your ITB from the hip to below the knee. Do for 1-2 minutes on each side of the leg.

<u>Shin Roll:</u> Place roller under your knees and slowly kneel down placing both shins on the roller. Slowly roll back and forth from bottom on the knee to the top of the ankle.

Core Workout Exercises

The "Core" is not just your abdominal muscles. This section focuses on the hips, abdominals, obliques, lower back, upper back, and shoulder girdle. The core is a system – not a set of abdominal muscles. When you exercise your stomach muscles, make sure to exercise and stretch your back and sides also.

<u>Advanced Crunch</u> - **(Legs up):** Lie on your back with your feet straight in the air. Keep your legs straight up in the air for the advanced crunches. Cross your hands over your chest and bring your elbows to your knees by flexing your stomach. ***Keep your feet on the floor if you prefer to make this exercise a little easier.***

Reverse Crunch: In the same position as the regular crunch, lift your knees and butt toward your elbows. Leave your head and upper body flat on the ground. Only move your legs and butt.

(Do not do if you have severe lower back injury or if this hurts your back)

Double Crunch: Lift hips and shoulders off the floor at the same time in one motion.

ight Elbow to Left Knee: Cross your left leg over your right leg. Flex your
omach and twist to bring your right elbow to your left knee.

eft Elbow to Right Knee: Cross your right leg over your leg. Flex your
omach and twist to bring your left elbow to your right knee.

icycles: This is a mix between opposite elbow to knee crunches with bicycling
your legs. Alternate from side to side for prescribed reps and do not let feet
uch the floor.

PT RESET

Some of my favorite exercises (that are easy to neglect) will help anyone build a stronger "core" and focus on the muscles that the sit up and crunches alone do not engage. The next series of exercises make up the PT RESET. Use it as a workout cooldown, warmup, or in between exercises as an active rest if you prefer.

<u>PT RESET - Swimmers:</u> Lie on your stomach and lift your feet and knees off the floor by flutter kicking repeatedly as if you were swimming freestyle – build up to 1:00 – or keep feet still but off the floor.

<u>PT RESET - Hip Rolls:</u> Lie flat on your back with your knees in the air as in the middle picture below. Keep your shoulders on the floor, rotate your hips and legs to the left and right as shown below.

PT RESET - Arm Haulers: Lie on your stomach. Lift your chest slightly off the floor and wave your arms from your sides to over your head for 30 seconds.

PT Reset - Reverse Push-ups - Lie on your stomach in the down push-up position. Lift your hands off the floor instead of pushing the floor. This will strengthen your upper back muscles that oppose the chest muscles. (Also called Hand Release portion of the **Army Hand release pushup**)

PT Reset – Birds: Lie on your stomach with your arms spread to the height of your shoulders. Lift both arms off the floor until your shoulder blades "pinch" and place them slowly in the down position. Repeat for 10-15 repetitions mimicking a bird flying.

PT RESET - Plank Pose and One Arm Plank: To complete the Crunch Cycle, try getting into the plank position and see if you can hold it for at least 1 minute. As you advance, lean on the left / right arm as you increase the time. Or do the plank in the UP Pushup position.

In fact, when you fail at pushups during the workout, stay in the UP - Pushup position for an extra 30-60 seconds each time. This will prepare you well for the long periods of time in the "leaning rest" as well as strengthen your body for crawling obstacles.

Practice the Plank more often now as many tests are dropping situps and adding the plank pose as part of the fitness test.

PT Reset - Dirty Dogs –In all fours position again, lift your right leg from the hip working the glutes to help balance the hip / ITB / thigh connections.

(Great for hip development)

PT Reset: Bear Crawls or Stair Crawls– Walk like a bear on all fours. This gets tough quickly. Think of this as a plank pose in motion.

Advanced Abdominal Exercises: Do not do if you are a beginner! These exercises are not ideal for weak or injured backs. If you cannot do the lower back exercise / plank pose exercises for 1:00 – do not attempt these exercises.

Tip to reduce strain on the lower back WITH LEG LEVERS, FLUTTERKICKS Lift your butt off the ground about an inch and place your hands underneath your butt bone, thus taking some of the strain off the lower back.

Flutter-kicks - Place your hands under your hips. Lift your legs 6 inches off the floor and begin walking, raising each leg approximately 36 inches off the ground. Keep your legs straight and moving. This is a four count exercise.

Leg levers - Lift your feet 6 inches off the floor. Raising both legs approximately 36 inches off the ground, keep your legs straight and off the floor until specified number of repetitions are complete.

Scissors – Lay on your back. Lift your feet 6 inches off the floor. Open and close both legs approximately 36 inches apart, keep your legs straight and off the floor until specified number of repetitions are complete.

eg Tuck – (aka Hanging knee ups) You can spice up your core work and even ▪place situps with this challenging exercise. Hang from the pullup bar and bring ⟩ur knees to your elbows. Grip and core work is critical to this one. The Army ⟩w does these exercises instead of situps for their PT tests.

Descriptions of the PT exercises

<u>Regular Push-ups</u> - Lie on the ground with your hands placed flat next to your chest. Your hands should be about shoulder width apart. Push yourself up by straightening your arms and keeping your back stiff. Look forward as you perform this exercise.

<u>Wide Push-ups</u> - From the same position as the previous push-up, place your hands about six to twelve inches away from your chest. Your hands should be greater than shoulder width apart. The slight change of the arm distance change the focus of what muscle are exercised.

<u>Triceps Push-ups</u> - From the same position as the regular push-up, place your hands under your chest about 1-2 inches away from each other. Spread your legs in order to help with balance. This exercise will concentrate more on the triceps of the arm than the chest.

Hand Release Pushups – The new changes the pushup exercise and adds the hand release to ensure pure and properly executed pushups. Plus, it adds in an upper back component to balance out the chest and front deltoid muscles. Do a regular pushup, then lift the hands off the floor in between reps.

Pull-ups (regular grip) - Grab the pull-up bar with your hands placed about shoulder width apart and your palms facing away from you. Pull yourself upward until your chin is over the bar and complete the exercise by slowly moving to the hanging position. Use assisted versions if needed.

Pull-ups (reverse grip) - Grab the pull-up bar with your hands placed about 2-3 inches apart with your palms facing you. Pull yourself upward until your chin is over the bar and complete the exercise by slowly moving to the hanging position.

*note – using reverse grip - keep your hands in and do not go wider than your shoulders

<u>Parallel Bar dips</u> - Grab the bars with your hands and put all of your weight on your arms and shoulders. Do not do these exercises with added weight, if you are a beginner, or if you have had a previous shoulder injury. **To complete the exercise, bring yourself down so your elbows form a 90 degree angle (no less of an angle) and back to the up position.**

Get good at pull-ups and dips as they will help you pull yourself up and over climbing obstacles when faced with a wall, rope, or ladder climb.

Mix in different grips for variety (wide grip, close grip and alternated grip). Note: When using a reverse grip, keep your hands in and do not go wider than your shoulders, as you will develop some elbow tendonitis similar to that of tennis elbow.

<u>When you fail at pullups, add in DB rows, assisted pullups or pulldowns to complete the set.</u>

Weightlifting Exercises Explained

Weight training exercises build muscle, joint and tendon strength needed for any contact sport. Preparing for some of the load bearing events require lifting, or at least a cycle of lifting / strength training focus.

Bench Press: Lie on your back on a bench, placing the legs bent with feet flat on the floor on both sides of the bench. Extend your arms upward, grab the bar or dumbbells just greater than shoulder width and lower the bar to your chest slowly. The bar should hit just below the nipples on your sternum. Extend your arms again to a locked position and repeat several times.

Pull-down Machine – This is an easier form of pull-ups, but you must start somewhere. Using a pull-down machine, grab the bar, sit down and pull the bar to your collar bones. **Change grips as you can on the pull-up bar (wide, regular, close and reverse).**

B rows: Grab a dumbbell (DB) in one hand and lean forward onto a bench, supporting your back with your opposite knee and hand. Pull the DB up to your chest, hold for 1 second and slowly extend the arm. Repeat 10/arm.

MJDB #1 - Multi-Joint Dumbbell Exercise: Perform a bicep curl, then press the dumbbells over your head with a military press, and then go straight into a triceps extension - repeat in reverse order to get to the starting position. **Option:** Go heavier and skip the triceps extension if you prefer.

1   2   3   4

Then repeat in reverse order 4,3,2,1.

PS- You can skip the triceps extensions if you prefer to go heavier on the squat, bicep, overhead press.

MJDB #2: Same as above but add in a squat when your hands are in the down bicep position (by your hips)

Same as MJDB#1 plus a squat / deadlift

MJDB #3: Same as MJDB #2 plus you add in a squat thrust and 1-5 push-ups. 1-5 push-ups is recommended per repetition.

Repeat in reverse order and continue MJDB#2

Thruster (front squat into over head press) – Explode upward from the front squat position straight into an overhead press or push press.

Thrusters with dumbbells – You can do these with dumbbells as well or even a single plate. The goal is to squat and forcefully stand and use the momentum of the upward movement to easily lift the weight over your head.

Farmer Walks – Work your grip and your core and simulate carrying boat handles on land with this exercise. Use 40-50lbs in a bag with a handle, dumbbell, kettlebell – BUT only in one hand at a time.

Dead Lift / Power Clean Starting Position - Side View - Keep your head up, back straight, and lift with your legs, not only your back.

Dead Lift – With the barbell on the ground, place feet about shoulder width apart and bend down to grab the bar as shown. Keep your back straight and your head upright. Pull the barbell to your hips by standing (straighten legs and keep hips forward). Use the legs and hips to lift the weight NOT YOUR lower back. **DO NOT DO THIS EXERCISE WITH HEAVY WEIGHT IF YOU HAVE NEVER TRIED THIS EXERCISE. Try the Kettlebells / Dumbbells dead lifts or the exercise MJDBs instead.**

Power Clean is one of the most dynamic exercises in athletics. Make this movement fast and get the momentum of the barbell moving fast from the start so it is an easy transition with the power relay into the torso / arms.

ang clean - Pull the barbell to your hips by standing (straighten legs and keep ɔs forward – dead lift). Use the legs and hips to lift the weight NOT YOUR wer back. Now swing the barbell to the chest by bending your knees and opping your waist 6-12 inches. Drop weight to your waist and repeat - DO 'ITH LIGHT WEIGHT BARBELL OR DUMBBELLS. (MJDBs for beginners to ɪrbell lifting)

ang Clean with Front Squat Option - as with the power clean the front squat optional but a great addition to all muscle groups. With the bar stopped at your ɑist. Slowly drop a few inches and explode as you would do with a power ɛan. Hang clean is a power clean that starts with the barbell at your waist.

Chapter Seven: The Lightweight Shoulder Workout

This shoulder routine is great for post rotator cuff shoulder surgery, and physical therapy patients. See link to video that explains all of the exercises in actual progression.

The Lightweight Shoulder Workout / Extra Lift Options

This can be done with lightweight dumbbells or food cans / water bottles. This shoulder routine is great for post rotator cuff / shoulder surgery physical therapy patients but will help build stability in the smaller muscles of the shoulder. See link to video that explains all the exercises in actual progression.

LATERAL RAISE: More than 5 pound dumbbells is not recommended for this exercise. Keep your shoulders back and your chest high. Lift weights parallel to ground in a smooth controlled motion, keep your palms facing the ground. Follow the next 6 exercises without stopping.

THUMBS UP: After performing 10 regular lateral raises, do 10 lateral raises with your thumbs up, touching your hips with your palms facing away from you and raising your arms no higher than shoulder height.

THUMBS-UP/DOWN: Continue with side lateral raises. As you lift your arms upward, keep your thumbs up. Once your arms are shoulder height, turn your hands and make your thumbs point toward the floor. Repeat for 10 times, always leading in the up and down direction with your thumbs.

FRONT RAISE - THUMBS-UP: Now, for 10 more repetitions, to work your front deltoids. Lift the dumbbells from your waist to shoulder height keeping your thumbs up and arms straight.

CROSS-OVERS: With your palms facing away from you and arms relaxed in front of your hips, bring your arms up and over your head as if you were doing a jumping jack (without jumping). Cross your arms IN FRONT of your head and bring them back to your hips for 10 repetitions.

<u>Bicep Curl – Military Press Combo</u> - Perform a bicep curl, then press the dumbbells over your head with a military press, repeat in reverse order to get to the starting position. Add in 5 shrugs every rep to top off shoulder workout. (Increase weight if you prefer)

Section Three: Workouts and Explanations

This section is to help explain some of the workout designs. The goal in these workouts is to do what you can or have time for. If you do not have a pool, try another form of non-impact cardio. If you have a pool but do not swim, try swimming some, but focus on the treading and dynamic stretching, as this is exceptional for your hips, legs, and lower back. You can also work your shoulders and elbows as well by doing jumping jacks, or other underwater movements with your arms to work your joints in a full range of motion.

Chapter Eight: About The Workouts Specifics

Warmup / Stretch
You will see a warmup of 5-10 minutes, which may include stretching at the start of your workouts. This can be whatever you prefer. You can do it with a bike, jog, walk or other quick cardio activity, or the squat or pushup pyramid, with short run warmup. Mixing in dynamic stretches in between sets during the 25 meter runs is another way to continue the warmup.

The PT / Circuit Workouts:

PT Pyramid Warmups - Find a place to do 15-25m of dynamic stretches in between exercises. Often, the burpee, squat, or pushup pyramids will be the warmup. Do 1 rep of exercise – run 25meters – do 2 reps, run 25m … Usually the pyramid will only go up to 5 or 10 sets. Or you can replace 25m jogs with walks or jumping jacks – 10 reps. A good place to do the short runs is a basketball court, tennis court or field. You do not have to repeat in reverse order down the pyramid unless it says to do so.

Circuit Workouts - You will see several different circuit routines in this workout program. Basically, a circuit workout is designed to move you as quickly through a workout as possible. There are no rest periods in a circuit until the end. Moving from one exercise to the other is the only rest you will get, but you will rarely be using the same muscle group two times in a row. So, there is actually rest built into the workout.

Warmup Pyramids - You will often see a warmup called Run and Pushups (or Squats) Pyramids at the top of the workouts. This means you find a place to jog or walk fast from one end of a room to another. We like to use a field or basketball / tennis court. Do 1 pushup or squat – run 25meters – 2 pushups or squats – run 25m – 3 pushups or squats … Keep going up to 5 or 10 sets and mix in some dynamic stretches during the 25m sections (buttkickers, frankensteins, side steps, high knees, side steps, etc.). Once you get to 10, you are done with the warmup. Usually, the set will be from 5-10 and depicted as such: Run / Pushup Pyramid 1-10.

Tabata Intervals - Do 20 second sprint / 10 second easy pace for timed sets in the workout, which is usually done on bike, elliptical, or rowing machines.

ife Cycle Workout – To ride a stationary bike with increasing resistance levels, ace bike on manual mode. Start off at level 1 or 2 and increase the resistance very minute until failure, and then repeat in reverse order. If your bike increases to 20 levels, increase resistance by 2 levels every minute. Otherwise, just crease by one level if bike tops out at 10-12 levels.

xtra Weekend Cardio - Over the course of Friday, Saturday, and Sunday, try accumulate _____ minutes (will progress each week) over the weekend. The ne can be completed with 10 minute walks after each meal, long walks with the bg, etc.

wim PT - Is a great way to squeeze in swimming and upper body PT into the ame workout. Simply swim the specified distances (usually 100 yards or eters), get out of the pool and do pushups, and abdominal exercises. Repeat is sequence at least 5-10 times.

ini-Mobility Day – For only two sets, do the following: 5 minutes of non-impact ardio activity and 5 minutes of stretching, foam rolling or massage tooling for a tal of 20 minutes. This is an excellent cooldown activity and you can shorten it extend it as desired.

T Reset – You will see this throughout the workouts days. Work to complete all a non-stop circuit.

T RESET:
everse Pushup20
irds -20
rm haulers-20
wimmers 1 min
ide plank 1 min (right) Plank 1 min
ide plank 1 min (left)

If you have access to a pool, consider Treading Water (video options)

Pool Mobility Day Off (full article)

Dry Land Mobility Day:

Best with nonimpact cardio options, do 5 minutes of easy cardio, followed by 5 minutes of stretching, foam rolling, or massage tooling and repeat 5 times for a total of 50 minutes (60 min with transitions).

Then, if available, get in the pool and do the following:

Tread water for 10 minutes - Work on big scissor kicks, breast stroke kicks, an arm range of motion strokes (like jumping jacks off the bottom of the pool).

Then, much like warming up with a variety of dynamic stretches before running: Try all dynamic stretches in the pool, in about chest-deep water (butt- kickers, Frankenstein walks, high knee lifts, leg swings (front / back / side to side).

> **Swim or tread water – 5-10 minutes**
> **Butt Kickers - 1 minute**
> **Frankenstein Walks - 1 minute**
> **High Knee / Hip openers - 1 minute**
> **Side Steps with hip opener - 1 min**
> **Leg Swings Front / Back - 1 minute**
> **Leg Swings (Left / Right) - 1 minute**
> *(Repeat with more options or longer time if needed)*

Butt Kickers - 1 minute: Jog slowly and flex your hamstrings to pull your heels to your butt on each step. Do with knees down then with knees up for 30-60 seconds.

Frankenstein Walks - 1 minute: Walk and kick high each step. Try to kick your hands in front of you. Do 10 kicks with each leg.

Bounding - 1 minute: Do high powered skipping for 1 minute. Start off with regular skipping then lift knees high each step. Do in place for 1 minute

Side steps w / hips openers - **30 seconds each direction:** Work lateral movement into the warm-up. Step sideways by lifting the leg and opening the hip to the side you step. Do for 1 minute back and forth alternating in each direction.

Leg swings – **1 minute:** Stand still and lift legs back and forth with legs straight at full range of motion of your hip (front / back). Then swing leg left and right in front of your body for 10 reps each leg.

Side Leg swings – **1 minute:** Stand still and lift legs back and forth with legs straight at full range of motion of your hip side to side (left / right).

The Program

This Tactical Fitness program will challenge you and may push you to failure many days. But there are recovery days built into the middle of the week on Day 3 or Day 4. You still want workouts that will push your perceived limits, but you need at least one day off per week (5-6 workouts / week), with one of those days being a Recovery Day. This is challenging, but not impossible. I promise you that you will be amazed at what you can do after you complete this twelve-week course. Do the stretches, foam rolling, dynamic warmups and water time for best results.

Running Replacement

During the beginning phases of ANY workout, some people need LESS running mileage when starting a workout plan. If you are finding the running / speed workouts to be too much, replace some of the runs with equal timed non-impact cardio events such as the bike pyramid, elliptical and rowing Tabata intervals, and swimming using the Running Non-Impact Replacement.

Good luck with the program and remember to consult your physician first before starting any program if you have not exercised in several months or years. If you need help with any fitness related questions, please feel free to email me at stew@stewsmith.com.

The Workouts

The charts below contain twelve weeks of workouts to help you rebuild that fitness foundation and better prepare for life after 40. The goal of starting after a long period of time without training—or if this is your first-time training—is to TREAT YOURSELF LIKE A BEGINNER. This is what Phase 1 is all about. Give it 21 days to build a new habit of easy fitness without getting too sore, injured, or burned out. Building a foundation of fitness is all about building a new habit of moving. Eventually this motivation to train will become a habit and your own discipline will drive the growth of your abilities.

ABOUT the 21 Day Habit Building Program:

Beginner Cycle: Days 1-21: Calisthenics / Weight Training Mix and Non-impact cardio.

- The goal here is the do some form of activity daily for these first 21 days – even if that is just walking for 10 minutes after every meal.

- In the 21 Day Chart, only repeat the exercises not separated by an underlined exercise. For instance:

Repeat 5 times
Pushups 5-10
Bicep curl/tricep ext–10
Shoulder workout
Walk / run/bike - 15:00

*You will only repeat 5 times the pushups, bicep curls, and tricep extensions for 5-10 reps each. You will only do the Shoulder Workout once and the walk, run, or bike for 15 minutes (once).

Weeks 4-6: Calisthenics and Weights Mix Foundation Building with Cardio (Running Optional)

Weeks 7-12: Transition into Calisthenics / DBs Only and Running and / or Non-Impact Cardio Progression

Enjoy the workout charts below. They will challenge you and help you perform like you did decades before:

The 21-Day Habit Foundation Building Program

Day 1	Day 2	Day 3
Crunch Cycle -10 each **Squats 25** total while walking up/down stairs Walk or bike 15:00	**Day 2** **Repeat 5x's** Pushups -10 / MJDB#1-10 Squats - 10 **Shoulder workout** **Walk or bike 15:00**	**Day 3** Crunch Cycle Circuit -10 **Mini-Mobility Day** **Repeat 3 times** Bike, row, elliptical 5 min Roam roll or stretch 5 min
Day 4 **Repeat 5 times** Pushups 5-10 Bicep curl/tricep ext–10 **Shoulder workout** Walk / run/bike - 15:00	**Day 5** **Crunch Cycle 10 each** **PT reset** Walk / run/bike - 15:00	**Day 6 Repeat 5x's** Walk / run/ bike - 4:00 squats - 20 / lunges - 10
Day 7 **Crunch Cycle Circuit -10** **Mini-Mobility Day** **Repeat 3 times** Bike, row, elliptical 5 min Roam roll or stretch 5 min	**Day 8** **Repeat 5 times** Jumping jacks - 10 Pushups - 10 (no rest) Shoulder Workout PT Reset	**Day 9** **Repeat 3 times** Walk or bike 5:00 squats - 20 lunge-10/leg
Day 10 **Crunch Cycle 15 reps** **Shoulder workout** Walk / run / bike - 15:00 **PT reset**	**Day 11** **Repeat 3 times** Plank pose – 1:00 Bench dips – 5-10 Walk or bike - 15:00	**Day 12 Repeat 5x's** Jumping jacks - 10 Pushups – 10 **Shoulder workout** Walk, bike 15-20 min
Day 13 **Crunch Cycle -15 reps** Squats – 3 x 15 reps Walk or bike - 15:00	**Day 14** **Repeat 4x's** jumping jacks - 10 Pushups – 10 **Shoulder Workout** **PT Reset**	**Day 15** Crunch Cycle Circuit -10 **Mini-Mobility Day** **Repeat 3 times** Bike, row, elliptical 5 min Roam roll or stretch 5 min
Day 16 **Repeat 5x's** MJDB#2 - 10 Squats - 10 / lunges 10 **Shoulder Workout**	**Day 17** **Crunch Cycle 15 reps** Walk or bike – 15-30 min PT reset	**Day 18** **Repeat 4x's** Pushups - 10 Squats –15 **Shoulder Workout**
Day 19 **Crunch Cycle 15 reps** Walk / run / bike – 15-30 minutes	**Day 20** **Repeat 5x's** Pushups - 10 Squats - 20/crunch- 20 Cardio of choice 20 min	**Day 21** **Crunch cycle 15 reps** **Squat 50 total** during walk or bike 20-30 minutes
*Every day – Stretch 10 minutes after exercise – head to toe		

Weeks 4-6: Calisthenics / Non-Impact

Spring - Week 4 – Calisthenics / Weights Mix – Running Optional		
Day 1	Day 2	Day 3
Upper body Workout Warm-up bike / walk - total 10:00 / Stretch **Repeat 5 times** jumping jacks 10 crunches 10 pushups 10 Light weight Shoulder **Repeat 3-4x's** Cardio - 5:00 - but make each minute harder than the previous (increase speed, resistance) MJDB#1 – 10 reps crunches - 25 pushups - 10-15 plank pose 1 min DB Rows - 10 reps Light weight Shoulder Walk/jog mix or bike, elliptical, rower, swim 15-20 minute cool-down Stretch	Lowerback plan – Core and Stretches Long Cardio / Legs Your choice - 45-60 minutes of any mix of bike, walk/run, or other cardio mixes - but every 10 minutes - stop and do 20 squats / 10 lunges **PT RESET:** Reverse Pushup 20 Birds -20 Arm haulers-20 Swimmers 1 min Side plank 1 min (right) Plank 1 min Side plank 1 min (left)	Walk or jog 5:00 light stretch Light weight Shoulder **Repeat 3 times** walk/jog or bike 5 min Bench press 10 military press 10 MJDB#1 - 10-15 rep DB rows 10-15 pushups 10-15 crunches 25 plank pose 1 minute Light weight Shoulder Walk/jog mix 15-20 minute cool-down Stretch

Week 4 - Calisthenics Weights Mix – Running Optional		
Day 4	Day 5	Day 6
Mobility Day **Repeat 5 times** Any non impact cardio (bike, elliptical, row, swim) 5 minutes Foam roll or stretch 5 minutes **If pool available:** swim 5 minutes tread 5 minutes dynamic stretches in water 5 minutes If no pool do stretches in the Lower Back Plan	Full body LWS - 5 lbs **Repeat 5 times** jumping jacks 10 squats 10 crunches 10 pushups 10 Pull / Leg Workout: **Repeat 3 times** pullups max OR DB rows 10/arm DB bicep curls 10/arm DB squats 10 **Repeat 5 times** jumping jacks 10 pushups 5-10 crunches 20 Push / Leg Workout **Repeat 3 times** Pushups 10-15 reps DB chest press 10 lunges 10/leg dips 10 MJDB#1 - 10 Lightweight shoulder Cardio Cooldown - 30 minutes of steady cardio - walk, bike, jog, etc...	Weekend walks – How much can you walk this weekend? Walk in the AM____ 10 min walks after meals _____ **PT RESET:** Reverse Pushup20 Birds -20 Arm haulers-20 Swimmers 1 min Side plank 1 min (right) Plank 1 min Side plank 1 min (left) Walk in the PM____ Can you get 1-2 hours worth of walking or other cardio options? And stretch 10 minutes each day over the weekend

Week 5 - Calisthenics / Weights Mix – Running Optional		
Day 1	Day 2	Day 3
Warmup with 1-10 Pushup pyramid - walk/jog 25yards do 1 pushup, walk.jog 25yds do 2 pushups...up to 10 / stretch. Lightweight shoulders **Repeat 3x's** MJDB#2 - 10reps crunches -25 pushups - 10-15 plank pose 1 min Squats 10 DB Rows - 10/arm **PT Reset:** Reverse Pushups 10 Birds 10 Arm Haulers 10 Walk 15-20 minute cool-down	Lowerback Plan **Long Cardio** Your choice - 45-60 minutes of any mix of bike, walk/run. **PT RESET:** Reverse Pushup20 Birds -20 Arm haulers-20 Swimmers 1 min Side plank 1 min (right) Plank 1 min Side plank 1 min (left)	Mobility Day **Repeat 5 times** Any non impact cardio (bike, elliptical, row, swim) 5 minutes Foam roll or stretch 5 minutes **If pool available:** swim 5 minutes tread 5 minutes dynamic stretches in water 5 minutes If no pool do stretches in the Lower Back Plan

Week 5 - Calisthenics / Weights Mix – Running Optional		
Day 4	Day 5	Day 6
Squat / pushups pyramid: squat 1 / pushups 1 run 25m. squat 2 / pushups 2 run 25m...keep going up until you fail at pushups - stop at 10. *do on basketball court, field, driveway etc..	Lowerback Plan Long Cardio Take a long walk or walk/run combo today - or bike for as long as you have time. 30min? 45min? 1 hour? plus?	Warmup with 5-10 min easy walk/jog Lightweight shoulders **Repeat 5 times** Jumping jacks 10 Pushups 5 Plank pose 15 secs Squats 10
Repeat 3 times Pushups max DB rows 10/arm Lunges 10/leg MJDB#2 - 10reps Situps or crunches 20	**PT RESET:** Reverse Pushup20 Birds -20 Arm haulers-20 Swimmers 1 min Side plank 1 min (right) Plank 1 min Side plank 1 min (left)	**Repeat 3 times** Military press 10 DB rows 10 Step up 5 / leg MJDB#2 - 10 Crunches 20 3 min fast / slow interval walk/jog OR NOT....just slow if needed.
PT Reset: Reverse Pushups 10 Birds 10 Arm Haulers 10 Walk 15-20 minute cool-down		Cardio Cooldown - 15 minutes of steady cardio - walk, bike, jog, etc...

Week 6 - Calisthenics / Weights Mix – Running Optional		
Day 1	Day 2	Day 3
Push, Pull, Core, Cardio Pushups Pyramid 1-5 - run 25m in between: 1 pushup - walk/run 25m, 2 pushups...stop at 5. **1 min sets TEST:** Pushups 1 min Pullups 1max - any? Situps 1 min or plank pose 1 min Cardio 5 min - How far do you get in 5 min of any cardio? **Repeat 3 times** Bench press 10 Pulldowns 10 Reverse Pushups 10 Birds 10 Arm Haulers 10 Cardio 5 min Lightweight Shoulder Walk, jog, swim, or bike 20 minutes for max distance.	Leg Day Squat pyramid 1-10 - run /walk 25m in btwn: 1 squat - 25m, 2 squats - 25m...stop at 10. For intermediate level: Squat pyramid 1-10 up/down flight of stairs: 1 squat - run up/down stairs, 2 squats up/down stairs...up to 10 - stop. **Repeat 3 times** Bike, walk, or row 3 min fast Leg ext 10 or lunges 10/leg Leg curl 10 or squats 20 (air) Leg press 10 (if available) or dead lift 5 How far can you bike, elliptical, or row for 15 minutes?	Cardio Day Pick one for 30 minutes of pick and choose combinations for 30-40 minutes total: Bike or walk, or walk/jog mix 15 minute warmup **15min of fast / slow:** 1 min fast / 1 min slow of the above choice of warm up. Or walk 10 minutes after every meal in your day if too busy **PT RESET:** Reverse Pushup20 Birds -20 Arm haulers-20 Swimmers 1 min Side plank 1 min (right) Plank 1 min Side plank 1 min (left)

Week 6 - Calisthenics / Weights Mix – Running Optional		
Day 4	Day 5	Day 6
Full Body	Mobility Day	**Cardio Weekend**
Warmup with 5 min cardio options / light stretch	**Repeat 5 times** Any non impact cardio (bike, elliptical, row, swim) 5 minutes Foam roll or stretch 5 minutes	Try to mix in 60-90 minutes spread through the weekend of some sort of movement: walk, jog, bike, elliptical, swim, or other form of movement.
Repeat 3 times Jumping jacks 10 pushups 5-10 Crunches 10-20 Squats 10	**If pool available:** swim 5 minutes tread 5 minutes dynamic stretches in water 5 minutes	Even if you break it up with 10 minute walks after meals or long walks of the dog. **Get out and move.**
Lightweight Shoulder **Repeat 3 times** Cardio 5 min Pushups 10 DB rows 10 Farmer walk up/down stairs 3x MJDB#2 - 10 Plank pose 1 min	If no pool do stretches in the Lower Back Plan **PT RESET:** Reverse Pushup20 Birds -20 Arm haulers-20 Swimmers 1 min Side plank 1 min (right) Plank 1 min Side plank 1 min (left)	
Cardio 15-20 min of walk, jog, bike, mix in a pyramid (every minute gets tougher with increase of resistance, incline or speed - start easy - end easy)		

Week 7-12: Calisthenics and Weights Progression / Cardio Options

Week 7 - Calisthenics / Weights Progression – Cardio		
Day 1	Day 2	Day 3
Pushup / Squat pyramid 1-5 warmup - run 25m 1 pushup / 1 squat, run 25m 2 pushups, 2 squats...keep going to 5/5. **Repeat 5 times** Jumping jacks 10 Pushups 5-10 Squats 10 **Repeat 3 times** Pullups max OR DB rows 10/arm Pushups or Db bench 5-10 Squats 10-20 (air) Lunges 10/leg crunches 25 plank pose 1 min Cooldown cardio 15-20 minutes of walk, bike, jog..etc, Your choice for max distance.	Cardio 20 min bike Pyramid - each minute is tougher than previous minute. IF AVAILABLE 20 min walk/run combo or walk longer if you prefer. **Upper Core** **Spread throughout day:** **Repeat 2 times** Reverse pushups 10 Birds 10 Arm Haulers 10 - Plank Pose 1 min Lower back plan - do it later in the evening **PT RESET:** Reverse Pushup20 Birds -20 Arm haulers-20 Swimmers 1 min Side plank 1 min (right) Plank 1 min Side plank 1 min (left)	Pushup / Squat pyramid 1-5 warmup - run 25m 1 pushup / 1 squat, run 25m 2 pushups, 2 squats...keep going to 5/5. **Repeat 3 times** Pushups 10-15 DB bench 10 Pullups - max? or DB rows 10/arm MJDB#2 - 10 Lighter Weight **Repeat 3 times** DB Military press 10 DB Squats 10 Light weight shoulders Cooldown cardio 15-20 minutes of walk, bike, jog..etc, Your choice for max distance.

Week 7 - Calisthenics / Weights Progression – Cardio		
Day 4	Day 5	Day 6
Mobility Day **Repeat 5 times** Any non impact cardio (bike, elliptical, row, swim) 5 minutes Foam roll or stretch 5 minutes **If pool available:** swim 5 minutes tread 5 minutes dynamic stretches in water 5 minutes If no pool do stretches in the Lower Back Plan	Cardio / Core 20 min bike Pyramid - each minute is tougher than previous minute. IF AVAILABLE 20 min walk/run combo on or just walk longer if you prefer. **Upper Core Spread throughout day:** PT RESET: Reverse Pushup20 Birds -20 Arm haulers-20 Swimmers 1 min Side plank 1 min (right) Plank 1 min Side plank 1 min (left)	**Warmup with 10 min run or bike** **Repeat 5 times** Walk or walk/jog combo 5 minutes Pushups -___? Pullups - ____? or DB rows 10/arm Squats 10-15 Light weight shoulders *Cooldown cardio 15-20 minutes of walk, bike, jog..etc, Your choice for max distance.* Lower back plan – stretches Try to get an extra 40 minutes of cardio this weekend – spread throughout the weekend.

Week 8 – Calisthenics / Weights Progression – Cardio		
Day 1	Day 2	Day 3
Warmup with 5 minute cardio of choice

Lightweight Shoulder

Repeat 3 times
jumping jacks 10
squats 10
pushups 10
pullups 3

Repeat 3 times
Bench Press 10 or
Pushups 15
Crunches 1 min

Repeat 2-3 times
Pulldowns 10
DB rows 10
DB Thrusters 10
Rev crunches 1 min
Lunges 10/leg

Repeat 3 times
Squats 10
Double crunch 1min
MJDB#2 - 10
Plank pose 1 min

Lightweight Shoulder

Follow with steady cardio of walk, jog, bike, swim, elliptical or any of your choice for 20 min | Faster Paced Cardio options mixed with higher resistance:

Walk/jog combo - walk 1 min jog 30-60 seconds as long as you can

Or bike - fast /slow for 40-60 total minutes

Stop two times during the cardio section and do:

Core:
crunches 10
rev crunches 10
double crunches 10
left crunches 10
right crunches 10
bicycle crunches 10

PT RESET:
Reverse Pushup20
Birds -20
Arm haulers-20
Swimmers 1 min
Side plank 1 min
(right) Plank 1 min
Side plank 1 min
(left) | Upper Body Plus Mobility Day

Repeat 5 times
jumping jacks 10
pushups 10
pullups 1-5

Repeat 5 times
bike, elliptical, row or swim 5 minutes
5 min stretch or foam roll

If pool
swim 5 min
tread water 5 min
dynamic stretches 5 min in chest deep water

OR

Follow with any cardio of your choice 10 minutes and dynamic / static stretches on land.

Repeat 2 times
Reverse pushups 10
Birds 10
Arm Haulers 10
Plank Pose 1 min |

Week 8 - Calisthenics / Weights Progression – Cardio		
Day 4	Day 5	Day 6
Faster Paced Cardio options mixed with higher resistance: Walk/jog combo - walk 1 min jog 30-60 seconds as long as you can **Or bike - fast /slow for 40-60 total minutes** Stop two times during the cardio section and do: **Core**: crunches 15 rev crunches 15 double crunches 15 left crunches 15 right crunches 15 bicycle crunches 15 plank pose 1 min Rev pushups 15 Birds 15 Arm haulers 15 Lower back plan (stretches only)- do it later in the evening	Push, Pull, Legs, Core Lightweight Shoulder **Repeat 2 times** 5 Min cardio Pushups 10-15 Pullups max DB rows 10 MJDB#2 - 10 reps **Repeat 2 times** 5 Min cardio Military press 15 DB bicep curls 10 DB squats 15 DB lunges 10 **Repeat 2 times** plank pose 1 min Pushups max crunches 25 Woodchopper squats 10 **Walk, jog, swim, or bike 10 minutes for max distance**	Faster Paced Cardio options mixed with higher resistance: Walk/jog combo - walk 1 min jog 30-60 seconds as long as you can **Or bike - fast /slow for 40-60 total minutes** Stop two times during the cardio section and do: **Core**: crunches 20 rev crunches 20 double crunches 20 left crunches 20 right crunches 20 bicycle crunches 20 plank pose 1 min Rev pushups 20 Birds 20 Arm haulers 20 Lower back plan (stretches only) - do it later in the evening

Week 9 - Calisthenics / Weights Progression – Cardio		
Day 1	Day 2	Day 3
Repeat 5 times Jumping jacks 10 Pushups 5-10 Plank pose 10 seconds **Repeat 2-3 times** Bench press 10 or Pushups max Pullups - max reps or DB rows 10 **Dips** - max MJDB#1 - 10 reps **Core Set:** crunches 15 rev crunches 15 double crunches 15 left crunch 15 right crunch 15 bicycle crunch 15 Reverse pushups 20 Birds 20 Arm haulers 20 Plank pose 1 min Lightweight Shoulders **Cardio Section:** 2 mile walk/jog mix OR row 10-20 min worth	5:00 warmup **Cardio / Leg Day Option:** Walk and/or jog mix 2 miles - every 5 minutes stop and do 20 squats or 10 lunges per leg. Bike, elliptical, row, or swim 20 min or walk 20 minutes Finish with Lowerback plan stretches only **PT RESET:** Reverse Pushup20 Birds -20 Arm haulers-20 Swimmers 1 min Side plank 1 min (right) Plank 1 min Side plank 1 min (left)	Mobility Day **Repeat 5 times** Any non impact cardio (bike, elliptical, row, swim) 5 minutes Foam roll or stretch 5 minutes **If pool available:** swim 5 minutes tread 5 minutes dynamic stretches in water 5 minutes If no pool do stretches in the Lower Back Plan

Week 9 - Calisthenics / Weights Progression – Cardio		
Day 4	Day 5	Day 6
Repeat 3 times jumping jacks 10 pushups 10 squats 10 stretch **Push Set x 2:** Bench press 10-15 or Pushups 10-15 DB tricep ext. 10 Dips - 10-15 Lightweight Shoulders **Pull Set x 2:** Pullups - max Pulldowns 10 DB rows 10 DB bicep curls 10 DB Rows 10/arm MJDB#2 - 10 reps **Leg Set x 2:** Squats 20 Lunges 10/leg WC Squats - 10 MJDB#2 - 10 Cardio option of choice 20 minutes	5:00 warmup **Cardio / Leg Day** Walk and/or jog mix 2 miles OR row 1000m Or Bike / elliptical or swim 20 minutes BUT - every 5 minutes stop and do 20 squats or 10 lunges per leg. Finish with **PT RESET:** Reverse Pushup20 Birds -20 Arm haulers-20 Swimmers 1 min Side plank 1 min (right) Plank 1 min Side plank 1 min (left)	Warmup 5 minutes Full Body Day **Repeat 5 times** Jumping jacks 10 Pushups 10 Plank pose 30sec. Squats 10 Pullups 1-5 **Repeat 3 times** Bench Press 10 Pulldowns 10 Thrusters 10 Abs of choice 20 **Repeat 2 times** DB rows 10 Lunges 10/leg Farmer walks up/down stairs 3x Cardio option of choice 20 minutes

Week 10 - Calisthenics / Weights Progression – Cardio		
Day 1	Day 2	Day 3
Warmup with 5 min cardio option of your choice - jog, walk, bike, elliptical, rower. **repeat 3 times** Jumping jacks 10 Pushups 10 Birds 10 **Repeat 3 times** Cardio 5 min Bench press 10 Pullups max Db rows 10/arm Pushups – max Abs of choice 25 Plank pose 1 min **Do 1-2 times throughout workout** Lightweight shoulders 5# MJDB#1 - 10 Cardio Interval: 1 min fast - 1 min slow for 20 minutes **PT Reset** Reverse pushups 20 Birds 20 Arm haulers 20 Plank pose 1 min	**Cardio / Leg Day** Add in squats 10-20 reps every 10 minutes of cardio time 40-60 minutes of your choice: swim, bike, row, elliptical, jog... or mix 2 x 30 min options or 2-3 x 20 min options of above or others. can you push to 75-90 minutes of cardio???	Mobility Day **Repeat 5 times** Any non impact cardio (bike, elliptical, row, swim) 5 minutes Foam roll or stretch 5 minutes **If pool available:** swim 5 minutes tread 5 minutes dynamic stretches in water 5 minutes **PT RESET:** Reverse Pushup20 Birds -20 Arm haulers-20 Swimmers 1 min Side plank 1 min (right) Plank 1 min Side plank 1 min (left)

Week 10 - Calisthenics / Weights Progression – Cardio		
Day 4	Day 5	Day 6
Calisthenics / Weights / Cardio Warmup with **Repeat 5 times** jumping jacks 10 Pushups 10 Reverse Pushups 10 **Repeat 3 times** Pullups max DB rows 10 Bench press 10 Plank pose 1 min Pullups max or Pulldowns 10 Pushups max Crunches 20 MJDB#1 - 10 Lightweight Shoulders Run 2 miles - for time-_____? or bike / elliptical / swim / rows 20 minutes	Cardio of your choice 60 minutes Note how far you get after 1 hour of walking, walking / running mix, backpacking, swimming, rowing, biking, or elliptical - your choice Divide 60 min through the day if you must..30 min in the am / pm **PT RESET:** Reverse Pushup20 Birds -20 Arm haulers-20 Swimmers 1 min Side plank 1 min (right) Plank 1 min Side plank 1 min (left)	Warmup with 5 minute cardio of choice **Repeat 3 times** Bench press 10-15 Crunches 1 min Pulldowns 10-15 Rev crunches 1 min **repeat 2-3 times** Squats 10-15 Double crunch 1min MJDB#2 - 10 DB Thrusters 10 Pick an upper body push, pull, leg, and full body exercise and complete the circuit 3 times resting with abs after each exercise Follow with steady cardio of walk, jog, bike, swim, elliptical or any of your choice for 20-30 min

Week 11 - Calisthenics / Weights Progression – Cardio		
Day 1	Day 2	Day 3
Warmup with 5 min cardio option of your choice - jog, walk, bike, elliptical, rower... **Repeat 5 times** Jumping Jacks 10 Pushups 5-10 **Repeat 3 times** Bench press 10 Military press 10 Tricep ext 10 Pullups max and/or Pulldowns 10 Bicep curls 10 **Repeat 3 times** MJDB#1 - 10 Dips 10 DB rows 10/arm Crunches 25 Plank pose 1 min **Pushups Pyramid** - 1-10 - run 25m 1 pushups, run 25m 2 pushups, run 25m 3...keep going to 10. Cardio cooldown 10 min or more of your choice. Easy pace.	Core / Cardio **Cardio / Core x 2** Crunches - 20 Cardio 2 minutes Rev crunch 20 Cardio 2 minutes Double crunch 10 toe touches - 10 Left crunches - 20 Cardio 2 minutes Right crunches 20 cardio 2 minutes Bicycle crunch 10 cardio 2 minutes plank pose 1 min Lower back plan - do stretches and core exercises **PT RESET:** Reverse Pushup20 Birds -20 Arm haulers-20 Swimmers 1 min Side plank 1 min (right) Plank 1 min Side plank 1 min (left)	Warmup With Non impact Cardio 5 min **Squat Pyramid** - 1-10 - run 25m 1 squat, run 25m 2 squats, run 25m 3...keep going to 10. 5 min bike or elliptical or rower **Repeat 3 times** 5 min tabata interval (20 sec sprint / 10 sec easy) on bike Squats 10 Lunges 10/leg no weight Farmer walk up/down stairs 2x Burn 100 calories burnout - how quickly can you burn 100 cals on any cardio machine? _____ or how fast can you run/walk 1 mile stretch legs

Week 11 - Calisthenics / Weights Progression – Cardio		
Day 4	Day 5	Day 6
Mobility Day	**Fullbody**	Core / Cardio
		Cardio / Ab
Repeat 5 times	**Repeat 3 times**	**workout x 2**
Any non impact	Cardio 5 min	Crunches - 20
cardio (bike,	Squats 10-20	Cardio 2 minutes
elliptical, row, swim)	Bench press - 10	Rev crunch 20
5 minutes	pullups max OR	Cardio 2 minutes
Foam roll or stretch 5	pulldowns 10,10	Double crunch 10
minutes	(wide, regular grip)	toe touches - 10
	crunches 20	Left crunches - 20
If pool available:	Burpee or pushup	Cardio 2 minutes
swim 5 minutes	pyramid 1-5: 1	Right crunches 20
tread 5 minutes	pushup run 25, 2	cardio 2 minutes
dynamic stretches in	pushups run 25	Bicycle crunch 10
water 5 minutes	...to 5 reps (or	cardio 2 minutes
	burpees)	plank pose 1 min
If no pool do		
PT RESET:	Lightweight	Lower back plan - do
Reverse Pushup20	shoulders	stretches and core
Birds -20		exercises
Arm haulers-20	**Repeat 3 times**	
Swimmers 1 min	MJDB#2 - 10	WEEKEND GOAL
Side plank 1 min	DB Rows 10/arm	
(right) Plank 1 min	Thrusters – 5-10	Long weekend
Side plank 1 min	Lunges 5/leg	cardio of your
(left)	crunches 20	choice - 60 minutes
		total
	Walk / jog 2 miles	
	or bike, row, swim 20	swim, bike, row,
	min	elliptical, jog...or mix
		2 x 30 min options or
		3 x 20 min options of
		above or others.

Week 12 - Calisthenics / Weights Progression – Cardio		
Day 1	Day 2	Day 3
Light weight shoulders	5:00 warm up stretch	Light weight shoulders
Repeat 5 times jumping jacks 10 pushups - 10	**Cardio / Legs / Core** Walk, bike, swim, elliptical - get 30 minutes of either or mix of two or more for more than 30 minutes.	**Repeat 3 times** jumping jacks 10 pushups - 10
Repeat 3 times Bench press 10-20 Pullups max Pulldowns 10		**Repeat 3 times** Bench press 10-20 Pullups max Pulldowns 10 Pushups 10 Bicep Curls 10 DB rows 10 MJDB#1 - 10
Repeat 3 times Pushups 10 Crunches 20 Reverse pushups 10 Birds 10 Arm Haulers 10 Plank Pose 1 min MJDB#1 - 10	BUT every 10 minutes stop and do Squats 20 Lunges 10/leg Plank pose 1 min	**Lift / Core Cycle x1** Crunches 20 Pulldowns 10 Rev Crunches 20 Military press 10 Double crunch 10 MJDB#1 - 10 Left Crunch 20 DB rows 10/arm Right crunch 20
Cardio Workout Tread or Swim 15-20 minutes or bike pyramid, elliptical or row Tabatas (20 sec fast / 10 sec slow for 15 minutes	**PT RESET:** Reverse Pushup20 Birds -20 Arm haulers-20 Swimmers 1 min Side plank 1 min (right) Plank 1 min Side plank 1 min (left)	

Week 12 - Calisthenics / Weights Progression – Cardio		
Day 4	Day 5	Day 6
Mobility Day **Repeat 5 times** Any non impact cardio (bike, elliptical, row, swim) 5 minutes Foam roll or stretch 5 minutes **If pool available:** swim 5 minutes tread 5 minutes dynamic stretches in water 5 minutes If no pool do **PT RESET:** Reverse Pushup20 Birds -20 Arm haulers-20 Swimmers 1 min Side plank 1 min (right) Plank 1 min Side plank 1 min (left)	5:00 warm up stretch **Cardio / Legs** Walk, bike, swim, elliptical - get 30 minutes of either or mix of two or more for more than 30 minutes. BUT every 10 minutes stop and do Squats 20 Lunges 10/leg Plank pose 1 min	Warmup with 5 min cardio of choice **Repeat 2 times** Bench press 10 Pulldowns 10 **Repeat 2 times** DB Rows 10/arm DB Thrusters 10 **Repeat 2 times** MJDB#1 - 10 Lightweight shoulder **Crunch Cycle x1** Crunches 20 Pulldowns 10 Rev Crunches 20 Military press 10 Double crunch 10 MJDB#1 - 10 Left Crunch 20 DB rows 10/arm Right crunch 20 **Weekend goal:** Walk 10-15 minutes after every meal or get in a 6th workout - Repeat any of the days of this week.

Lose the Body Fat / Inches

Going from a highly active job with required morning workouts and bi-annual fitness tests, to retirement or a desk job can often lead to quick and steady weight gain if you do not either continue the physical activity or learn how to eat like a person who does significantly less activity. Far too many people who change jobs or retire seem to forget how active they were prior to retirement and still eat like a highly active person. It does not take long for this error to yield a twenty-pound weight gain. This can happen in as little as a year, and in fact often does. So, I think the first goal when you make a drastic change to your activity level is to make sure you tackle the food intake immediately. It becomes more and more difficult to out-work your diet, and when you reach military retirement age, it is nearly impossible. So, you have to hit your healthy weight and fitness from both ends: Calories IN and Calories OUT.

Ideas for the Calories IN Side of the Equation:

Make a list of EVERYTHING - Everything you eat, snack on, and drink all day long needs to be put on paper so you can see it, and do the math. Add up the calories / portion sizes of every meal, snack, and drink. Also keep track of water intake. In fact, add more water (typically). PERSONAL CATCH: This was life changing. I realized I liked to eat a spoonful of peanut butter as a snack throughout the day. This is not an "unhealthy" snack, but does add significant calories. A few days a week, I was adding 800 calories to my day with a few servings just because it was there. This adds up by the end of the week and was my main contributor to maintaining / slowing gaining a pound a month. No more peanut butter in the house and I dropped five pounds in 2 weeks!

Be Smart - There are many Weight Loss Myths out there that many have tried with mixed short-term but horrible long-term results. If you are starting to gain weight, avoid these myths.

Eat Smart - Think about what goes into your body. It does not take an advanced education to realize that Ho-Ho's and soda are going to wreck your calorie intake and provide very little nutrients.

Eating plan - This eating plan will help your body keep the metabolism high and burn calories throughout the day. Limiting calories of processed sugar and other processed foods, adding fiber, and adding protein will help lean you out quickly and in a healthy manner.

Some Foods Should be Avoided and All Need to be Controlled - As you age trying to outwork your diet becomes a thing of the past. Your ability to consume more calories is easier but the ability to burn them off at higher rates is more difficult. I have found that it came down to more ***portion control*** versus what I was eating. I do not eat sugar snacks, drink sodas, or sugary drinks. Instead eat a modest portion of chicken, steak, fish and nuts. These are high calories foods that are great for the body. However, controlling that urge to eat more has been the ticket to not gaining five pounds a year. If you are still hungry after dinner, and there is still more food just sitting there, save it for tomorrow. Try to top off your meal with a salad or extra glass of water.

Making a Plan of what you will eat each week will keep the discipline in your world that you may lack in retirement. After all, it is easy to work out for an hour a day, but keeping poor food choices out of your mouth the other 23 hours requires real motivation and discipline.

Get Out and Move to Get the Calories OUT:

The other half of the fitness and health equation is to keep moving. This can be done through a large variety of movements and activities.

Keep up your activity - If you enjoy exercising as a daily habit, keep it up, but play around with new training ideas and figure out roughly how many calories you are burning in a workout session. You can add in other outdoor activities like walking the dog, yard work, or any other active hobby you enjoy.

You may need to up your game a bit and add a second activity session into your day. If you are an early bird exerciser with a higher metabolism in the morning, that is great, but you may find that your afternoons are sluggish. This is especially true if you eat a big lunch followed by little activity. Now, a quick walk /jog of the dogs, a swim for 20 minutes, or a bike ride helps after a smaller meal to stay awake and productive at work, and burning more calories in the day.

Exercise - Keeping a daily PT program in retirement is a must, but it does not have to be anything you use to hate about military PT tests or standards. Some people like to "be all you can be" and still keep up with the Army PT Standards of running, pushups, and situps. I would recommend replacing situps with plank poses for a better core activity, but other calisthenics like pushups, dips, and pullups are great additions to any PT program and can be easily done at home.

Some form of cardio - Maybe by now, daily running has taken its toll on your knees or back. Perhaps replacing running with bike, elliptical, or rowing machines or swimming will be something to do riding into retirement. If you still like to run, consider running every OTHER day, while mixing in non-impact options on the days in between running.

Non-Impact Cardio workouts - 4-5 times a week of 45-60 minute sessions of cardio exercise: elliptical gliding, walking, jogging, swimming, rowing, or biking are great examples of how to burn calories. If you are overweight and need to lose over 50 lbs., I do not recommend running. Select a non-impact form of the aerobics listed above.

Stay Limber - If you sit too long during the day, you will start to ache. Get up and stretch. Check out the Lower back Plan for starters to stay limber and keep the core tight. But, consider yoga or other stretching and mobility programs to keep the joints working at full range of motion.

Get out of the house - Get to the gym for access to pools and equipment, and to be around other fitness-focused people. Play sports like pickle-ball, racquetball, and tennis if you are into competition and moderate to low levels of challenge. Get hardcore if you wish and try weight lifting contests or races if your joints can still handle it. The point is, have fun with your fitness and use it as a social outlet as well.

See Links: Nutrition | ABDs of Nutrition | Lean Down

Gaining weight later in life (40 years and over) can be as easy as looking at food for most of us. Losing it however is much tougher than it was in our twenties. Men and women both have a decrease in metabolism after forty years old, and some even earlier. We can however, fight the effects of aging with a daily exercise plan, stretching, de-stressing, and eating foods that are rich in protein, carbs, fats, vitamins, and minerals.

In closing, find out where the leaks are in your diet by keeping track of food coming in and see if you can add something to your exercise plan that burns more calories (higher intensity, duration, resistance training, etc). Avoid sugar and focus on foods that keep you full and that are higher in fiber and vitamin rich nutrients as listed in the links above. Good luck. Time to get to work!

The Complete Tactical Fitness Series

As a military, police, and fire fighter fitness writer for over 20 years now, the term *Tactical Fitness* did not exist when I started. Now, in the last decade resources have been spent by all groups of tactical fitness and a new fitness genre has been born. The following is my current library of Tactical Fitness Programming to include books, ebooks, and online coaching products and services:

Tactical Fitness - At the core of this program is the Tactical Fitness Test which measures 12 standards for your physical capacity, including: cardiovascular conditioning, strength, muscle coordination, and stamina. Tactical fitness means having the skills needed to save lives and extend the limits of your endurance whether you are in the military, police, firefighting professions, or just an everyday hero. Also featured in the Tactical Fitness Test called the Dirty Dozen.

Tactical Strength - Tactical Strength is the lifting program used by Stew Smith and his Military, Police, Fire Fighter fitness program called the Heroes of Tomorrow. It is designed to build strength in the upper body, legs, and core to prepare you better for any load bearing activity (rucking, boat carry, log PT, etc). We also use the Tactical Strength Test to test elements of speed, agility, and strength / power.

Tactical Mobility is a comprehensive fitness guide for greater mobility, flexibility, and performance—designed for the men and women serving in military, special ops, law enforcement, emergency services. Tactical Mobility is a perfect fit for any fitness program as a stand alone "Mobility day" supplemented into your regular routine and will help you reach the pain free level of fitness. Gaining flexibility and mobility is the goal of the program and it will help with performance and help reduce injuries.

Tactical Fitness 40+ Series

Things to Consider As You Age

As we age, there are a few truths that every Tactical Athlete Over Forty must realize:

1 – **You cannot outwork your diet**. Typically, portion control is the answer, but depending on your goals, eating to gain weight is too easy. Eating to lose weight is more challenging after 40. Gone are the days of your twenties when you could eat whatever you wanted, train hard, and not gain weight. Eat less.

2 – **Add Mobility.** Before workouts, dynamic stretches and warmups are required. After a workout, stretching and some mobility work is recommended. But, once a week, a tough workout should be exchanged for a Mobility Day when needed or even when not needed.

3 – **Daily Running.** If you are a bigger person or you are feeling the pain of a life well-lived after 40, you may want to consider running every OTHER day. But on the days in between pick a non-impact cardio option. If you can end each day with swimming and a quick dynamic stretch session in the water, you will be amazed at the results – especially during higher mile running / load bearing workout cycles.

In a world where fitness can be the difference of life and death, we will be older for a longer period than we were younger. Learning how to progress into those decades smartly with added longevity training - typically in the form of active recovery days and mobility days is going to increase your abilities and decrease your pain. The following series is a new programming focused on an often-neglected age group of active duty and retired veterans of the tactical professions who need to rebuild and take their fitness to the next level in order to enjoy the latter half of their lives:

Tactical Fitness (40+) Foundation Rebuilding - Recovery from Injury or Inactivity (Part 1). This new beginner plan forces you to "treat yourself like a beginner." Even if you do not feel like it, giving yourself a few weeks to easily work your way back into the weight room or any fitness program will pay off and help you rebuild after a long period of inactivity.
Book | Ebook | Amazon Kindle / Paperback

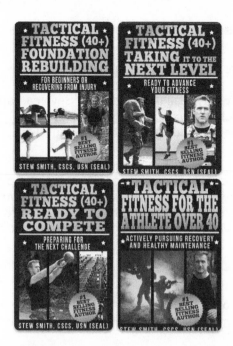

ctical Fitness (40+) - Taking It To The Next Level (Part 2) - Are you ready to dvance your fitness level? Well, *Taking It To The Next Level* after *Rebuilding e Foundation* (Part 1) is what this 12 week program is all about. Are you eady to Advance Your Fitness?
ok | Ebook | Amazon Kindle / Paperback

ctical Fitness (40+) - Ready to Compete - (Part 3) (Intermediate / Advanced vels) – After you have progressed through the previous phases, you may be ady for something new. Maybe a new challenge or "up your game" to a level at pushes you physically, but also focuses on stress relief and recovery after ugh workouts.
ok | eBook

ctical Fitness For The Athlete Over 40 - Actively Pursuing Recovery and aintenance - This is part 4 of the above series that is rather advanced but still cused on adding in an easy day and / or mobility day to the week as a way to cover in the middle of the week. This will enable for a better workout number 5, or 6 as the week moves into the weekend. Running every OTHER day with n-impact cardio will reduce stress on the knees. Use of non-impact cardio and imming pool for mobility is helpful as well. Book | Ebook | Amazon Kindle / aperback

Closing Remarks

Open Invitation - FREE Workouts!

We do local training for FREE in the Annapolis / Severna Park MD area year round. Our weekly schedule can be found at the Heroes of Tomorrow page. Check in with us prior to attending and fill out the questionnaire on the page above.

If you find this book helpful, let others know. You can also purchase multiple copies at a reduced price from our printer service if you have a large group of people who would benefit from this information. For any info on bulk purchases contact us at the email listed below for price savings per multi-book purchase.

ONLINE COACHING

Also if you need personal training help, check out the StewSmithFitness.com website where you can train with me through the Online Coaching program.

GOOD LUCK

Thanks for choosing a profession of serving your country. It is an honorable profession that requires commitment to stay fit and healthy so you can best perform your duties, to stay alive, and keep others alive.

Good luck with the program and remember to consult your physician first before starting any program if you have not exercised in several months or years. If yo need help with any fitness related questions please feel free to email me.

Contact us at stew@stewsmith.com if you need to ask questions about training, this specific workout, or you would like to attend our local workouts, make bulk purchases, or considering online coach

Made in the USA
Coppell, TX
28 June 2024

34056575R00059